Patient Safety

RESEARCH INTO PRACTICE

Patient Safety

RESEARCH INTO PRACTICE

Edited by Kieran Walshe and Ruth Boaden

Open University Press

Open University Press
McGraw-Hill Education
McGraw-Hill House
Shoppenhangers Road
Maidenhead
Berkshire
England
SL6 2QL

email: enquiries@openup.co.uk
world wide web: www.openup.co.uk

and Two Penn Plaza, New York, NY 10121–2289, USA

First published 2006

Copyright © Kieran Walshe & Ruth Boaden 2006

A catalogue record of this book is available from the British Library

ISBN-10: 0 335 21853 9 (pb) 0 335 21854 7 (hb)
ISBN-13: 9780 335 218530 (pb) 9780 335 218547 (hb)

Library of Congress Cataloging-in-Publication Data
CIP data applied for

Typeset by RefineCatch Limited, Bungay, Suffolk
Printed in Poland by OZ Graf. S.A. www.polskabook.pl

Contents

List of contributors

Anthony J. Avery, DM FRCGP, Head of Division of Primary Care, University of Nottingham, UK

Maureen Baker, DM FRCGP, Special Clinical Adviser, National Patient Safety Agency, London, UK

Paul Beatty, PhD C.Eng FIPEM, Senior Lecturer, Division of Imaging Science and Biomedical Engineering, University of Manchester, UK

Ruth Boaden, MA, MSc, PhD, Senior Lecturer in Operations Management, Centre for Public Policy and Management, Manchester Business School, UK

Tanya Claridge, BNurs (Hons) RGN, RHV, School of Psychological Sciences and Stockport NHS Foundation Trust, University of Manchester, UK

Gary Cook, MB ChB LLB MRCP FFPH, Clinical Effectiveness Unit, Stockport NHS Foundation Trust, UK

Caroline Davy, BSc, M Clin Psychol, C Psychol, Consultant Clinical Psychologist Research Fellow, Clinical Safety Research Unit, St Mary's Hospital, UK

Susan Dovey, MPH, PhD, Director, RNZCGP Research Unit, Dunedin School of Medicine, New Zealand

Aneez Esmail, MRCGP, MFPHM, PhD, Professor of General Practice Division of Primary Care, University of Manchester, UK

Rachael Finn, Research Fellow, Institute for the Study of Genetics and Biorisks in Society, University of Nottingham, UK

Martin Fletcher, Performance Manager, World Health Organization, World Alliance for Patient Safety, Geneva, Switzerland

Sally Giles, Research Associate, Institute of Medicine, Law and Bioethics, University of Liverpool, UK

John Hickner, MD, MSc, Professor of Family Medicine, Pritzker School of Medicine, The University of Chicago, Chicago, USA

Rachel Howard, BPharmHon, MRPharmS, DipClinPharm, Research Pharmacist, Nottingham Primary Care Research Partnership, Broxtowe and Hucknall Primary Care Trust, UK

Amanda Howe, MA, MD, MEd, FRCGP, ILT(M), Professor of Primary Care, Institute of Health, University of East Anglia, UK

Michael Jones, Professor of Common Law, Liverpool Law School, University of Liverpool, UK

Susan Kirk, PhD, MSc, BNurs. Senior Lecturer, School of Nursing, Midwifery and Social Work, University of Manchester, UK

Rebecca Lawton, PhD, Senior Lecturer in Health Psychology, Institute of Psychological Sciences, University of Leeds, UK

Martin Marshall, MSc, MD, FRCP, FRCGP, Head of Division of Primary Care, Professor of General Practice, National Primary Care Research and Development Centre, University of Manchester, UK

Caroline J. Morris, BPharm, MSc, PhD, MRPharmS, Research Fellow, Drug Usage and Pharmacy Practice Group, School of Pharmacy and Pharmaceutical Sciences, University of Manchester, UK

Dianne Parker, PhD, Professor of Applied Social Psychology, School of Psychological Sciences, University of Manchester, UK

Shirley Pearce, BA, MPhil, PhD, Director of Institute of Health and Centre for Interprofessional Practice, University of East Anglia, UK

Robert L. Phillips, Jr., MD, MSPH, Director, The Robert Graham Center, Policy Studies in Family Medicine and Primary Care, Washington, DC, USA

Stephen Rogers, MRCGP, MFPHM, MSc, Department of Primary Care and Population Sciences, Royal Free and University College Medical School, University College London, UK

Sally Taylor-Adams, BSc (Hons) PhD, Head of Incident Investigation, National Patient Safety Agency, London, UK

Richard Thomson, Director of Epidemiology and Research, National Patient Safety Agency, and Professor of Epidemiology and Public Health, Newcastle upon Tyne Medical School, UK

Charles Vincent, Smith and Nephew Foundation, Professor of Clinical Safety Research, Imperial College London, UK

Kieran Walshe, PhD, BSc (Hons), DipHSM, Professor of Health Policy and

Management, Centre for Public Policy and Management, Manchester Business School, UK

Justin Waring, PhD Research Fellow, School of Sociology and Social Policy, University of Nottingham, UK

Alison Watkin, BA, (Hons) Research Associate/Educational Facilitator, Centre for Interprofessional Practice, University of East Anglia, UK

Fiona Watts, BSc, (Hons) Centre Coordinator and Coordinator of Post-Registration Programme Centre for Interprofessional Practice, University of East Anglia, UK

Elizabeth West, PhD Lecturer and Post-Doctoral Fellow, London School of Hygiene and Tropical Medicine, London, UK

Maria Woloshynowych, BSc, PhD, Lecturer in Clinical Safety, Imperial College London, UK

Preface

Patient safety has moved from being a small and insignificant issue, of interest only to a few self-selected enthusiasts, to a position high on the agenda for managers, policy-makers and the public, in less than a decade. With prominent newspaper headlines about killer bugs, dangerous doctors and damaging drugs, the public and politicians are more aware than ever that healthcare organizations are not safe places to be. The pressure to do something to make healthcare safer, perhaps even as safe as other industries, is considerable. The challenge for all concerned is – what to do? How do you make hospitals, clinics and healthcare provision safe for patients? What needs to change to make care processes less error-prone, more consistent, less risky, and more safe? This book, on patient safety research and its impact on practice, hopes to provide at least some of the answers.

The idea for this book on patient safety research and practice came directly from the first meeting of the Manchester-based patient safety research network, one of several such networks which were set up in 2003 and funded jointly by the Medical Research Council, the Economic and Social Research Council and the Engineering and Physical Sciences Research Council. The Manchester network is focused on patient safety in primary care, and has over 100 members from academic, policy and healthcare provider backgrounds across the UK and internationally. It is a very eclectic and multidisciplinary group, and is hosted by Manchester's Institute of Health Sciences. When we held our first meeting in 2004, we quickly realized that having brought together some of the leading researchers and commentators on patient safety, we had a great opportunity to capture and spread some of their thinking and discussion, through an edited book. It quickly became apparent that while there were some books on risk management or patient safety, none seemed to do the two things we thought were most important: (1) to focus on researching patient safety issues and providing a rigorous empirical foundation for policy and practice; and (2) to bring together researchers and practitioners to share and debate research findings.

Producing an edited book like this is not always an unalloyed pleasure for the editors – when contributors don't write what you asked them to, or what they said they would, or don't deliver on time, or write far longer or shorter than you expected.

However, it is a tribute both to the professionalism and enthusiasm of our authors, and to the efficiency with which the editing process has been managed that this book emerged almost painlessly, and that we met our deadlines. Alas, little of the credit for the latter achievement is really due to either of us. We owe a huge debt to Rebecca Jones from the Institute of Health Sciences and Amy Bevell from the Centre for Public Policy and Management at Manchester Business School, who between them have managed this idea from inception to manuscript and beyond.

Kieran Walshe and Ruth Boaden
Manchester Business School
April 2005

Introduction

Kieran Walshe and Ruth Boaden

Until about ten years ago, patient safety was not an issue for debate, discussion or action by healthcare organizations, health systems, and policy-makers, nor was it the focus for much research. Clinicians had known – and perhaps accepted too readily – for at least 40 years that hospitals were hazardous places, where patients often suffered avoidable harm (Barr 1955; Moser 1956; Schimmel 1964; McLamb and Huntley 1967). The advance of medical technology had brought new therapies with great clinical benefits, but also with greater potential for harm. As the pace and complexity of clinical processes increased, the margin for error reduced. For patients, hospitals, clinics and other healthcare organizations had become more and more dangerous places to be. But in the public consciousness, there was little if any awareness of the uncertainties of and variations in healthcare delivery, and a somewhat naïve faith in the ability of the healthcare professions and institutions to provide consistent, high quality care.

It was the Harvard Medical Practice Study in the late 1980s, since replicated in Australia, New Zealand, the United Kingdom and elsewhere, which provided the first explicit empirical assessment of the harm done to patients by healthcare organizations and made manifest the scale and extent of the problems of patient safety (Harvard Medical Practice Study 1990). It found that almost 4 per cent of all patients admitted to hospital suffered an adverse event, and that 28 per cent of all adverse events were due to negligence. Thus, 1 per cent of all patients suffered a negligent adverse event during their admission. While most adverse events resulted in minimal or transient disability, 14 per cent caused or were implicated in the patient's death (and 51 per cent of these were judged to be negligent). But it was not until an influential report from the Institute of Medicine in 1999 brought the issue to widespread public attention in the United States that the problems of patient safety began to be taken seriously. Extrapolating from the Harvard study and other research which has suggested that between 3 per cent and 17 per cent of patients suffer some unintended harm, it concluded that there were 98,000 deaths due to medical error per annum in the USA, making medical error a more common cause of mortality than many high profile diseases (Institute of Medicine 1999). Policy-makers in the USA and in many other countries have responded with a raft of initiatives intended to tackle what has been described as the hidden epidemic of medical error and iatrogenic harm (Department of Health 2000, 2001). Governments have, often for the first time, invested substantial resources in building an infrastructure to identify, learn from and prevent adverse events and errors, and to establish programmes of research into patient safety (Shojania et al. 2001; NPSA 2004).

But using terms like 'epidemic' prompts misleading and unhelpful comparisons between medical error and patient safety and major clinical disease groups such as cancer, heart disease or stroke. While the consequences of each – in terms of patient morbidity and mortality – may be compared, the causes, processes, and approaches to dealing with them are very different. Errors and adverse events are fundamentally organizational – not clinical – in their aetiology. While clinical epidemiology can provide (as it did in the Harvard study) a vital empirical understanding of the incidence and characteristics of error and patient harm, it does not help us to understand the causes of error, when they so frequently relate to issues such as communication, teamwork, care process design, instrumentation and facilities, human resources, service organization, management, and leadership. A range of disciplines, including psychology, sociology, clinical epidemiology, quality management, technology and informatics, and the law all have important parts to play in analysing errors and adverse events, and they bring different and complementary theoretical frameworks and conceptual understandings of patient safety problems. A whole spectrum of methods and approaches to investigating and improving patient safety problems is available – such as incident reporting, claims review, database analysis, ethnographic observation and critical incident analysis – and each can be applied in different service areas, different specialties, and different health professions. Patient safety is not the province of any one discipline, research design or method of measurement, and real understanding and improvement in patient safety require a collaborative synthesis of these different perspectives and contributions.

This book provides a forum in which these different traditions and ideas are brought together, with the intention of promoting collaborative multidisciplinary approaches to patient safety research. Our aim has been to provide a broad introduction to the emerging field of patient safety research, and its contribution to policy and practice. The book cannot – and does not – set out to be a comprehensive or complete account of research into patient safety issues. As has already been noted, recent government investment has led to something of an explosion of new research, in what is now a fast developing field. Rather, our intention is to offer a coherent understanding of the main research traditions and key methods, in a form which should be useful both to the research community interested or involved in undertaking research and to the practitioner and policy-maker communities who are best placed to identify research needs and who are expected to translate research findings into practice. This latter connection – between research and practice – is often poorly made in other areas of health services research (Walshe and Rundall 2001). As a result, research activity is not well linked to real research needs, and research findings are inadequately disseminated and, at best, those findings are rather slowly taken up and used to influence practice, while, at worst, they are simply ignored. It is vital that patient safety research does not become disconnected from the needs and interests of healthcare organizations and patients, and is undertaken in ways that involve and take account of those interests. Fundamentally, it is in both researchers' and practitioners' interests to undertake good, rigorous, relevant research which makes a real difference to patient safety.

Overview of the book

Part 1 of the book (Chapters 1 to 6) presents a series of different theoretical or disciplinary perspectives on patient safety and explores what each can contribute to our understanding of errors and adverse events. First, in Chapter 1, Aneez Esmail offers a clinician's view of the challenges of patient safety, which emphasizes the extent to which doctors and other clinicians must learn to live with and tolerate the uncertainties of clinical practice – but notes that such tolerance can easily tip over into a complacent and self-serving acceptance of errors and adverse events. Then Elizabeth West explores the sociology of organizations in the context of safety in Chapter 2, Dianne Parker and Rebecca Lawton in Chapter 3 review the considerable contribution of psychology to the study of error and safety in healthcare, Ruth Boaden describes the development of quality management and its links with patient safety in Chapter 4, Paul Beatty provides a technological and informatics perspective in Chapter 5, and Michael Jones closes Part 1 of the book in Chapter 6, which examines the legal dimensions of patient safety.

Part 2 of the book (Chapters 7 to 13) presents a series of chapters focused on different approaches to measuring, evaluating or researching patient safety. It starts with John Hickner et al. exploring in Chapter 7 the development of taxonomies of patient safety – systems for categorizing, labelling and classifying errors and adverse events which are needed to make measurement and analysis reliable and meaningful. Then, in Chapter 8, Sally Giles et al. review the development of incident reporting systems in other industries and in healthcare, and consider what makes for effective systems of incident reporting. Tony Avery et al. then show in Chapter 9 how large existing databases of patient information, and data from processes such as chart review, can be used to research patient safety, drawing on a series of examples concerning prescribing and pharmaceuticals. Stephen Rogers et al. next tackle the use of critical incident analysis techniques, examining a range of approaches to investigating patient safety incidents and understanding their causation and consequences in Chapter 10. Then, in Chapter 11, Charles Vincent et al. explore the value of claims data – information about cases of clinical negligence litigation – to patient safety, reviewing studies of closed claims and examining the circumstances in which such data are useful tools for patient safety research. Next, Rachel Finn and Justin Waring in Chapter 12 explain how ethnographic approaches to researching patient safety can provide a richer and more nuanced understanding of patient safety issues, and their relationship to organizational culture and context. Finally, in Chapter 13 Susan Kirk et al. tackle the safety culture of organizations, and examine a number of tools which have been developed and used to measure or assess cultural aspects of patient safety.

Then, in Part 3 (Chapters 14 to 16) a number of case studies of improvement in patient safety are presented, which draw on the preceding theoretical and methodological contributions and are intended to show patient safety research in action, contributing to real improvement. In Chapter 14, Amanda Howe shows how patient safety issues are increasingly tackled in the education and development of healthcare professionals. Dianne Parker et al. examine the use of patient pathways and guidelines as tools for defining care processes and improving patient safety in Chapter 15, and Shirley Pearce, Fiona Watts et al. use Chapter 16 to explore the way that work to improve clinical team communication and functioning impacts on patient safety.

From these apparently divergent and quite different contributions there emerge some clear areas of congruence, and some interesting contrasts in approach. In Chapter 17 we return to the issues of what we can learn collectively about how we research and understand patient safety issues, and what the future agenda for researchers, policy-makers and practitioners could be. But some themes which run through a number of chapters in the book are worth raising here too, in this Introduction.

First, do we think about patient safety from our perspectives as individuals – doctors, nurses, managers, therapists, and so on – or do we see patient safety as primarily an organizational concern? How much are errors or adverse events the result of individual failures, or how much are they a property of the system within which the individual works? Most of our contributors emphasize the importance of the system or the organization as a determinant of patient safety, and play down the extent to which individuals should be made accountable for errors which result from a toxic organizational culture, poor process design or inadequate management systems. However, as Aneez Esmail's contribution in Chapter 1 makes clear, there is a long-standing and deeply entrenched belief among clinicians – and perhaps especially among doctors – in individual responsibility for decision-making and for clinical care. It could be argued that clinicians see themselves as independent practitioners, working within a system, rather than as part of that system. And, given the considerable freedom and autonomy that clinicians still enjoy, and the relative absence of systems of management or oversight for much of clinical practice, perhaps they are right to do so. But what does that mean for theoretical frameworks and models which focus on the organizational dimensions of patient safety, and pay rather less attention to issues of individual behaviour or culpability? How well do such models and frameworks fit the distinctive organizational structures and cultures of healthcare institutions?

This leads neatly to our second issue, which is, to what extent can healthcare organizations learn from or adopt the safety practices of other industries? How transferable are systems for incident reporting, investigation protocols, culture measures and other tools from one organizational context to another? There is a case for saying that healthcare organizations are different in fundamental ways which make such transfers more problematic. For example, one difference is the extent to which healthcare organizations are dominated by the professions, who have enormous formal and informal power and whose capacity to influence decisions and shape care processes is enormous. A second difference is the very limited extent to which what might be called the production processes in a healthcare organization are ever defined, made explicit, and documented. In most other manufacturing or service industries, a great deal of effort would be invested in standardizing these processes, so that their results were consistently acceptable. Yet few hospitals could provide an explicit account of what happens even to the most common patient groups, such as those admitted for heart attacks or strokes. Because the processes of care are often difficult to discern, identifying safety problems and taking action to improve safety are almost certainly harder in healthcare organizations. A third – and crucial – difference is the close and complex interrelationship between what might be called disease-harm and process-harm in healthcare organizations. In almost no other industry is it quite normal (or even sometimes desirable) for a consumer to die during their interaction with the service provider, yet this is exactly what happens in healthcare organizations. Distinguishing between morbidity and mortality problems which are generated by the system of care and those which result from the underlying progression of disease is always difficult. For healthcare organizations, the omnipresence of what we have called disease-harm makes it much more difficult to distinguish or prioritize what could be called process-harm – mortality or morbidity resulting directly from the way that care has been provided. Health professionals and institutions can all too easily become inured to errors or adverse events, and be too ready to reach for externalizing explanations for such occurrences rather than examine whether they result at least in part from the process of care. For these and other reasons, it seems that there are some grounds for arguing that healthcare organizations are exceptional entities in cultural and contextual terms, with some distinctive behaviours and structures which make simply transferring safety systems from another setting rather problematic. Of course, it is too easy to construct and hide behind an argument of healthcare exceptionalism, and it does not necessarily follow that these differences are always material considerations when transferring ideas or methods for improving safety from one context to another, but they do need to be taken into account.

Third, how much have healthcare organizations got to change if they are to reach the standards of safety which are attained in other industries? Or to put this another way, just how much scope for improvement is there in patient safety? We think that healthcare organizations have never really been designed to prevent or protect against errors, and our safety standards are far behind those in other sectors. It is clear from a number of contributions to this book that other industries place a much higher premium upon reliability or even upon the absence of error. So-called 'high reliability organizations' in areas such as air travel, banking, nuclear power, oil production, and so on have often invested many years of effort in developing an organizational culture and reporting structures that validate and emphasize the importance of safety. In contrast, healthcare organizations have no such tradition or established culture, and almost no track record in designing care processes to maximize patient safety and minimize error. Patient safety has been an implicit rather than an explicit concern, somewhat taken for granted by healthcare organizations and rarely figuring on the agendas of senior leaders and policy-makers. It has not been a vital concern to the organization, and if we are honest, patient safety failures have rarely had consequences for healthcare organizations or those who lead them. We should not underestimate just how much the healthcare environment and healthcare organizations need to change if they are to address this rather woeful record.

It was noted earlier that researchers, particularly those involved in the Harvard Medical Practice Study and its replications in other countries, have already played an important part in making patient safety a high priority in many countries, by providing empirical evidence of the harm done to patients in healthcare organizations. The new challenge is to use research to find ways to reduce or prevent that harm, and to improve the safety and quality of care. We said at the outset that we think no one discipline or research tradition owns the territory of patient safety, and that the best research – and the greatest improvements in patient safety and the quality of care – will result from the collaboration between researchers in different fields and practitioners. We hope this book will play some part in that endeavour.

References

Barr, D.P. (1955) Hazards of modern diagnosis and therapy: the price we pay, *Journal of the American Medical Association*, 159(15): 1452–6.

Department of Health (2000) *An Organization with a Memory: Report of an Expert Group on Learning from Adverse Events in the NHS*. London: The Stationery Office.

Department of Health (2001) *Doing Less Harm*. London: The Stationery Office.

Harvard Medical Practice Study (1990) *Patients, Doctors and Lawyers: Medical Injury, Malpractice Litigation and Patient Compensation in New York*. Boston, MA: Harvard College.

Institute of Medicine (1999) *To Err Is Human: Building a Safer Health System*. Washington, DC: National Academy Press.

McLamb, J.T. and Huntley, R.R. (1967) The hazards of hospitalisation, *Southern Medical Journal*, 60(5): 469–72.

Moser, R.H. (1956) Diseases of medical progress, *New England Journal of Medicine*, 255(13): 606–14.

National Patient Safety Agency (2004) *Research and Development Strategy 2004*. London: NPSA.

Schimmel, E.M. (1964) The hazards of hospitalisation, *Annals of Internal Medicine*, 60(1): 100–10.

Shojania, K.G., Duncan, B.W., Wachter, M.D. and MacDonald, K.M. et al. (2001) *Making Health Care Safer: A Critical Analysis of Patient Safety Practices*. Rockville, MD: Agency for Healthcare Research and Quality.

Walshe, K. and Rundall, T. (2001) Evidence based management: from theory to practice in healthcare, *Milbank Quarterly*, 79(3): 429–57.

PART 1
Perspectives on patient safety

1

Clinical perspectives on patient safety

Aneez Esmail

What is a clinical perspective on patient safety? Is there something clearly defined within the clinical process that improves our understanding of patient safety? Or perhaps is it the case that we have to define more clearly what the specific issues and problems are, so that others can give their perspective? In writing this chapter, I have taken the view that it is useful to set out the problems related to patient safety that I encounter as a clinician and let the reader judge, after reading other perspectives, how a deeper understanding may improve the problems that I have identified. In particular, I will bring the perspective of a family physician.

Uncertainty and general practice

As a clinician I take part in activity which is inherently unsafe. What I mean by this is that every day I make decisions and do things where the potential for something going wrong is significant. I am interested in patient safety issues because I recognize that a lot of what I do can result in harm to patients. However, I also know that if I draw on contributions from disciplines such as human factors research, sociology and psychology, I can gain a better understanding of why things go wrong and can develop safeguards to prevent this happening.

I have found that general practice or family practice, as it is known in many other countries, is in a way a strange and disturbing business. Quite frequently the stakes are high, especially when I think about what can go wrong. I can miss diagnosing a cancer in a patient with disastrous consequences. One day, a child may come to see me with flu-like symptoms and I will provide reassurance and paracetamol only to find out later that they may have meningitis. I prescribe drugs for patients that have the potential to cause horrendous side effects. I oversee the care of patients that is dependent upon near perfect communication between different providers. Every day, I deal with situations that have the potential for serious error and could cause harm to the patient. Externally it might seem that I do this with an air of confidence brought about by the apparent knowledge and experience that I have as a member of the medical profession. But scratch below the surface of what I do and you will see the doubts and mistakes, failures as well as successes and how uncertain and messy it all is.

Most of my patients come to me because I think they expect an orderly field of knowledge and procedure. Perhaps it's because of the way that medicine sells itself; perhaps it's the way that medicine is portrayed in the media and in documentaries. It all seems so certain, but the truth is, it isn't. Medicine isn't a perfect science, knowledge is constantly changing, information is uncertain, and, worst of all, the individuals who practise it are fallible. Of course, there is a science to the practice of medicine but so much of it happens because of habit, intuition and guesswork. Medical uncertainty is one of the core characteristics of medical culture and understanding its origins and its impact is an important component of the clinical perspective on patient safety.

Rene Fox in her research carried out in the 1950s (Fox 1957) has provided the still dominant description and analysis for considering how training for uncertainty takes place in medical practice. She describes three categories of uncertainty that medical students encounter. These are: (1) the limitations and gaps in medical knowledge; (2) the incomplete mastery of medical knowledge; and (3) the difficulty in differentiating between personal ignorance and limitations in medical knowledge. She describes how medical students have to decide what proportion of the huge body of knowledge needs to be mastered. They need to accept and recognize that they can never know all medical knowledge and that there is an irreducible minimum of uncertainty inherent in medicine. They also learn that much of practice is experimental and therefore a great deal of practice is provisional. In order to cope with this uncertainty, they develop certitude which is reinforced by observing how their teachers deal with uncertainty. The consequence of this training for uncertainty is that when things go wrong there is a tendency to concentrate on process and blame oneself or patients. This is summarized in Figure 1.1.

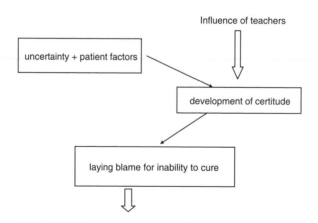

Figure 1.1 Training for uncertainty

The complexity of general practice

Karl Weick and Kathy Sutcliffe (2001) described what the particular problems were on an aircraft carrier when they were studying the features of high reliability organizations. They described how complex and dangerous the aircraft carrier was in terms of how it had to function and how it was staffed. General practice is nothing like an aircraft carrier but it can seem just as hectic, just as dangerous and I have paraphrased their description of what it is like on the deck of an aircraft for general practice (Box 1.1).

Of course it is not like this every day but it is not surprising that the world that I practise in is so potentially full of areas where things can go wrong. James Reason in his book *Human Error* (2003) describes how our propensity for certain types of error is the price we pay for the brain's remarkable ability to think and act intuitively, to sift quickly through the vast amounts of sensory information that constantly bombard us without wasting time trying to work through every situation anew. Systems that allow human imperfection present what Reason calls latent errors – errors waiting to happen (more details about this concept are given in Chapter 3).

Medicine and general practice, in particular, teem with examples of latent errors; writing out a prescription, which is a rote procedure that relies on my memory and attention is inherently unreliable. Inevitably I will sometimes specify the wrong dose or the wrong drug. Even when the prescription is written correctly, there is a risk that it will be misread. Another example is the procedures that we have developed for use in our practice when there is an acute emergency. I am absolutely certain that if we had a cardiac arrest in our practice, even though we have the right systems in place, there is still a chance that something would go wrong and there is a huge risk of a

---

Box 1.1 A day in the life of a general practitioner

Imagine that it is always a busy day and the whole of primary care has been shrunk to one room with one entrance. Patients come every ten minutes, wanting to be seen without having to wait too long. The waiting room is full and stuffy and children are crying and you know that if you run late, tempers will fray. Any kind of illness may present in a person of any age, physical as well as mental conditions; many patients do not speak the language of the doctors and reception staff. Some are drug addicts, some are alcoholics, and some are severely mentally disturbed, posing a real physical danger to the staff. Then impose severe constraints on the time available for diagnosis and investigation. The access to diagnostic aids is limited; everything you find out has to be on a basis of careful history taking and on the clinical examination, which frequently cannot tell you much because invariably patients present quite early in their illness. Now add a few cases of severe illness, people with multiple chronic problems and give me ten minutes to decide what is wrong. Make sure that I have no time to find out or to ask anyone any questions, ensure that I get interrupted periodically by phone calls and requests for home visits and make sure that any time that I have to find out about things after the consultation is finished is tied up with administration. Oh, and by the way, make sure that I am always right, always courteous and always safe.

mishap occurring. Everything that we do in terms of our workload, our chaotic environment, our team communication is all full of latent errors waiting to happen.

How does one cope with such uncertainty? With meticulous techniques, with continuous efforts to ensure that my knowledge is always up to date and that I always think of every possibility, I need never make an error. So when things do go wrong and I misdiagnose something or I fail to diagnose something, then it is easy to say that the error was avoidable. The reality is that I am almost certain to miss a diagnosis of cancer or of meningitis at least once in the course of my career. Cognitive psychologists and industrial error experts have demonstrated that we can reduce errors by strengthening processes and reducing reliance on people. We are taught that systems and structures are important, but it is difficult in my field to give up the belief in human infallibility. Every time I see a patient, I convince myself that I will offer the best treatment, drawing on my knowledge and my diagnostic skills. It is not vanity and I would argue that it is a necessary part of good medicine. It is true that things can go wrong quite easily sometimes but it is also true that effort does matter; diligence and attention to detail can make a difference.

This is why it is not surprising that many doctors take exception to talk of 'systems problems', 'continuous quality improvement' or 'process re-engineering'. That is the dry language of structures, not people. I am no exception; something in me demands an acknowledgement of my autonomy and therefore my ultimate culpability. Good doctoring is all about making the most of the hand that you are dealt. It is true that systems can be designed to reduce error. The reality is, no matter what measures are taken, doctors will sometimes make mistakes. It's not reasonable to ask doctors to achieve perfection. However, what is reasonable is that we never cease to aim for perfection and that we take personal responsibility for the errors that we do make.

What happens when things go wrong

It is important to understand how doctors think about and deal with medical mishaps because this might explain the approach that we take to medical errors. It offers another interesting perspective on clinical error.

Medical thinking about mishaps is deeply embedded in medical culture. I have already described how the key feature of medical practice and of general practice, in particular, was uncertainty. One of the consequences of training for uncertainty is the development of the culture of blame, with blame usually being placed on oneself but sometimes on the patient and even on others. One way of dealing with uncertainty is to concentrate on process, rather than on the result of the process. If one is doing the right thing, then theoretically one is practising competently.

What happens when doctors do make mistakes? Marilynn Rosenthal (1999) has gathered data on what happened in more than 200 specific cases of physicians with problems, ranging from physicians with barbiturate addiction to cardiac surgeons who continued operating despite permanent cerebral damage from a stroke. Rosenthal found a disturbing consistency in what happened. First, it usually took months, even years, before colleagues took effective action against a bad doctor, irrespective of how dangerous the problem might have been. Rather than a conspiracy of silence, Rosenthal describes the dominant reaction as uncertainty, denial, dithering and feckless intervention.

One particularly relevant example was from the recently completed Shipman Inquiry. Harold Shipman was a British general practitioner who was convicted of killing 15 of his patients. A subsequent Public Inquiry found that he was responsible for the deaths of 218 patients. I was the medical adviser to the Inquiry. One of the cases that we investigated was most unusual. Mrs Renate Overton was a 47-year-old asthmatic. One evening in February 1994, she had an asthma attack and called Shipman to visit her at home. He treated her with a nebulizer and the asthma settled. He gave Mrs Overton an overdose of diamorphine and waited until she had gone into respiratory and cardiac arrest before he called her daughter who was in the house to summon an ambulance. He went through the charade of attempting to resuscitate her until the ambulance arrived. When the ambulance arrived, Mrs Overton was, to all intents and purposes, dead. However, the paramedics were able to resuscitate her. Mrs Overton was taken to hospital and lived, for 14 months, in a persistent vegetative state. Shipman told the hospital staff that he had given Mrs Overton 20mgs morphine; he wrote in her medical records that he had given her 10mg of diamorphine, because she had begun to complain of chest pain. The medical staff realized that Mrs Overton was in the vegetative condition because of the morphine and that, because she was asthmatic, Shipman should not have given her any morphine at all, let alone 20mg. However, no one challenged his method of treatment or sought to investigate the circumstances of her admission. They assumed that it was a genuine mistake, but it was such unusual treatment that at the very least they should have instituted an investigation. Senior physicians were aware of the significance of the error yet kept their thoughts to themselves and did not take it further. If they had, Shipman might have been discovered and many further deaths could have been prevented.

Rosenthal's work gives us an understanding of why Shipman's medical colleagues took no action. Figure 1.2 summarizes what Rosenthal describes as 'There go I but for the grace of God' syndrome, with its resultant clubbing together of doctors, covering for each other, rather than being open about problems.

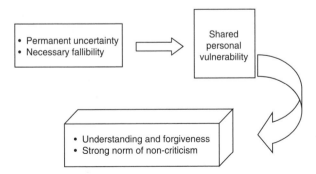

Figure 1.2 'There go I but for the grace of God' syndrome

Interestingly, there are well-described signs that can be identified before problems become established. Kent Neff, a psychiatrist working with problem doctors in America, is quoted in Gawande (2002) as describing four types of behaviour sentinel events. These are: (1) persistent poor, out of control or abusive behaviour; (2) bizarre or very erratic behaviour; (3) transgression of professional boundaries; and (4) a disproportionate number of lawsuits or complaints. Neff has also collected information on the causes of the problem. Most doctors turned out to have psychiatric illnesses, depression, bipolar disorder, drug or alcohol addiction and sometimes even outright psychosis. Others were struggling with stress, divorce and grief.

From the public point of view, this means that doctors who make mistakes should not be stigmatized as sociopaths but as human beings who are struggling with day-to-day problems. The difficulty is whether, once the doctor is rehabilitated, the public will be willing to be treated by a recovering drug-addicted general practitioner, a cardiac surgeon who is recovering from bipolar depression or a paediatrician who doesn't know the limits of his or her professional work. How much should the public know about past misdemeanours of physicians or about serious errors that have taken place? It is not the purpose of this chapter to articulate this debate but an understanding of why things go wrong is critical to any discussion about what happens afterwards, when the rehabilitation (if any) takes place.

However, because there is a pervading culture of blame and persecution, doctors get away with things that in situations of more openness, would identify the problem doctors and would protect patients. The culture will not change unless we are prepared to accept some sort of rehabilitation of people's lives and careers, and this is an issue for doctors as well as patients.

What are the implications in terms of research?

Our own work (Esmail et al. 2004) has found that, within primary care, problems with diagnosis account for the vast majority of claims for negligence. However, the problem of misdiagnosis is not unique to general practice. There has been a huge amount of work on understanding the problem of misdiagnosis, much of it related to how often findings from autopsies differ from the perceived cause of death. In a recently published book *Complications*, Atul Gawande (2002) provides a useful summary of the problem of misdiagnosis. Studies in 1998 and 1999 show that in nearly 40 per cent of cases, autopsies turn up major misdiagnosis in a cause of death. A review of autopsy studies concluded that in about a third of the misdiagnoses, patients would have been expected to live if proper treatment had been administered. What is even more surprising is that the rates at which misdiagnosis had been detected in autopsy studies have not improved since the 1930s. So despite all the recent advances in imaging and diagnostics, it appears that we seem to get the diagnosis wrong in at least two out of five patients who die. The point is that many errors do not get picked up and we are unaware of the many things that go wrong. So finding out how to improve things can be problematic especially if we do not even know the extent of the problem.

Gawande (2002) describes the Harvard study that looked at how often autopsies picked up misdiagnosis in the 1960s and 1970s before the advent of CT ultrasound and nuclear scanning and other technologies and then again in the 1980s after those technologies became widely used. Surprisingly, there was no improvement in these rates. The Harvard researchers found that regardless of the medical progress, physicians missed a quarter of fatal infections, a third of heart attacks and almost two-thirds of pulmonary emboli in the patients who died. It wasn't that the technology had failed, but rather that physicians did not consider the correct diagnosis in the first place. So we come back again to the problem of dealing with uncertainty. So understanding and dealing with uncertainty, especially in relation to the work of physicians, are important areas that need to be researched.

A classic essay written in 1976 by Gorovitz and MacIntyre explored the nature of medical fallibility, and postulated three reasons as to why there was so much uncertainty in medicine. One was ignorance: perhaps science affords only a limited understanding of how things happen. Second was ineptitude: the knowledge is available but as doctors we have failed to apply it correctly. Within the context of error, both of these are surmountable causes of error. The third possible cause, however, is insurmountable and they termed it 'necessary fallibility'. What this means is that there are some kinds of knowledge that science and technology will never deliver. When we ask science to move beyond explaining how things generally behave to predicting exactly how a particular person will behave, then perhaps we are asking for more than it can do. Each patient is quite unique. This is the necessary fallibility inherent in medicine. In some respects it is unpredictable, in others, with enough science and careful probing, it is entirely predictable. Of course, there is still room for improvement but it seems that there will always be things that doctors will get wrong. The core predicament of medicine is uncertainty. With everything we know about people and diseases and how to diagnose and treat them, it is difficult, especially for non-physicians, to understand how deeply this uncertainty runs.

The acknowledgement of medical error as a distinct entity and the development of a body of knowledge related to patient safety have highlighted the extent of the problem. We have just begun to understand the systemic frailties, technological faults and human inadequacies which are the cause of many medical mistakes. We know that even where there is knowledge of what is the right thing to do, we still fail to do it. There is no doubt that the contribution from sociologists (see Chapter 2), human factors research (see Chapter 3) and the other disciplines that are described in this book have helped our understanding of the problems. What is also clear is that all this knowledge has not made its way far enough into the practice of medicine. Work done in primary care, for example (Campbell et al. 2001), shows a huge variation in the adoption of guidelines (see also Chapter 15). A lot of medicine and general practice still lacks the basic organization and commitment to make sure that doctors do what they should be doing. Organizational structures are still not sufficiently developed to ensure that when effective guidelines have been set up that there is a mechanism which includes the appropriate dissemination and reward structures to ensure that they are incorporated into everyday practice. Even the monitoring of the implementation of many guidelines is frequently lacking. But the reality is that there is still abundant uncertainty over what should be done in many situations. The grey zones always occur when we consider problems related to specific individuals because there is frequently lack of clear scientific evidence on what to do (see Box 1.2)

Box 1.2 Examples of grey areas

- In patients with chest infections, a common problem in general practice, who should be referred to hospital and who should be treated at home?
- Which patient with back pain should be referred to surgeons?
- Which child who is feeling feverish and a bit off and has a rash, should be referred to hospital or sent home on antibiotics?
- Which patients with headache need further investigation?
- How should tiredness and lethargy be investigated by family physicians?

In many cases the answers are obvious, but sometimes we just don't know. In the end, in the absence of guidelines and evidence, we make decisions based on previous experience and judgement. Even where guidelines do exist, they frequently do not help us in making decisions about individuals. The work by Jack Wennberg (Wennberg and Gittelsohn 1982) on physician practice variation shows that the uncertainty at work, the varying experience, habits and intuitions of individual doctors can lead to very different care for people.

Neuro-psychology research has shown us how human judgement is prone to systemic mistakes. We over-estimate dangers, resort to learnt behaviour and do not handle lots of sources of information and data very well. Our judgement is affected by the order in which information is presented and how problems are framed. We are also affected by emotions and other extraneous factors and even by the time of day. We have an ability to recognize the right thing to do sometimes not because of a calculated weighing of all options but because of an unconscious form of pattern recognition.

It is not surprising that despite all the training and experience we doctors have, we are still prone to these fallibilities. This was well summed up by David Eddy (1984) who showed how many decisions made by physicians appear to be arbitrary, highly variable and with no obvious explanation. The implication of this arbitrariness is that for some patients it represents 'sub-optimal or even harmful care'. In some areas of clinical medicine, uncertainty can be reduced by group decision. But the idea of a group decision also runs counter to everything that doctors believe about themselves as individuals and about their personal ability to negotiate with patients on the best course of action.

In relation to patient safety, the challenge is to do research which will reduce the amount of uncertainty, not necessarily on new drugs or operations or new technology but on the small but critical everyday decisions that patients and doctors make. However, we also have to accept that a great deal of uncertainty about what we do will always remain.

In areas such as primary care, many of us work in isolated practices in the inner sanctum of the consulting room. With our imperfect science, what we as doctors want most is the opportunity where one's know how, ability or just gut instinct can come together to change the course of someone else's life for the better. In the actual situations that present themselves however, the situations when we do make the right diagnosis, when we do identify the child with meningitis and get it right, we can recognize that our efforts succeed. They don't always succeed but they do so often enough for us to continue in the way that we do. Perhaps that is the reason that doctors are so resistant to change.

Box 1.3 Key points

- The practice of medicine is inherently unsafe and will always be so.
- Doctors are trained to cope with uncertainty, with the consequence that when something does go wrong, they tend to focus on process and blame either themselves or the patients.
- Medical thinking about what happens when things go wrong is embedded in medical culture, and results in the profession clubbing together to provide support and maintain the norm of non-criticism.
- There are warning signs about things going wrong but there is also a need for the acceptance of rehabilitation of doctors after errors.
- The depth of uncertainty in the practice of medicine is not easily understood by those outside the profession and leads to different care for different people.
- Research from other areas has not made enough impact on the practice of medicine.
- The challenge is to do research which reduces uncertainty about the small but critical decisions made every day by doctors, while accepting that uncertainty will remain.
- Perhaps doctors are resistant to change because they get things right too – and this is where their efforts succeed in doing good.

References

Campbell, S.M., Hann, M., Hacker, J., Burns, C., Oliver, D., Thapar, A., Mead, N., Gelb Safran, D. and Roland, M.O. (2001) Identifying predictors of high quality care in English general practice: observational study, *British Medical Journal*, 323(7316): 784–7.

Eddy, D.M. (1984) Variations in physician practice: the role of uncertainty, *Health Affairs*, 3: 74–89.

Esmail, A., Walshe, K., Vincent, C., Fenn, P., Firth-Cozens, J., Elstein, M. and Davy, C. (2004) *Learning from Litigation: Using Claims Data to Improve Patient Safety*. Final report submitted to Department of Health, MCHCM, University of Manchester. Available from www.mbs.ac.uk/mchm.

Fox, R. (1957) Training for uncertainty, in R. Merton, G. Reader and P. Kendall (eds) *The Student Physician: Introductory Studies in the Sociology of Medical Education*. Cambridge, MA: Harvard University Press.

Gawande, A. (2002) *Complications: A Surgeon's Notes on an Imperfect Science*. New York: Picador.

Gorovitz, S. and MacIntyre, A. (1976) Toward a theory of medical fallibility, *Journal of Medicine and Philosophy*, 1: 51–71.

Reason, J. (2003) *Human Error*. Cambridge: Cambridge University Press.

Rosenthal, M.M. (1999) How doctors think about mishaps, in M. Rosenthal, L. Mulcahy and S. Lloyd-Bostock (eds) *Medical Mishaps: Pieces of the Puzzle*. Maidenhead: Open University Press.

Shipman Inquiry. Results available at http://www.the-shipman-inquiry.org.uk/fifthreport.asp

Weick, K.E. and Sutcliffe, M. (2001) *Managing the Unexpected: Assuring High Performance in an Age of Complexity.* vol 1. San Francisco: Jossey-Bass Inc.

Wennberg, J.E. and Gittelsohn, A. (1982) Variations in medical care among small areas, *Scientific American,* 246: 120–35.

2

Sociological contributions to patient safety

Elizabeth West

The sociological perspective

This chapter is an attempt to access the wider sociological literature on the organizational sources of safety and danger to determine the extent to which knowledge from this field can be used as a framework for research on adverse events in healthcare settings and quality improvement more generally. Concern about the frequency with which adverse events occur continues to rise (Vincent 1997). Adverse events occur in hospitals for many reasons. Some may be unavoidable. An uncommon allergic reaction to a properly prescribed and administered medication, for example, is unfortunate but is part of the risk associated with accepting any medical intervention. Some adverse events are the result of mistakes or malfeasance on the part of individuals. It is easy for an individual clinician to misread a prescription or administer the wrong dose of a drug to a patient as a result of stress or a momentary lapse of concentration. There are few occupations where errors and accidents are more costly than in health care. The list of mistakes that each clinician accumulates is probably some complex function of length of time in clinical practice, situational factors, individual characteristics, and random chance. Stories about staff causing deliberate harm to patients are rare but memorable and form an important constituent of public discourse about risk and danger in healthcare settings.

However, a sociological perspective suggests that many adverse events that occur in hospital are due to failures of the system rather than individual failures. Many of the errors, accidents, and disasters that happen in hospitals are rooted in features of the organization (Leape 1997). Starting from the premise that complex organizations have both the capacity to achieve goals that individuals cannot achieve and to introduce new sources of error, this chapter argues against automatically ascribing errors in organizations to the ignorance, incompetence, or immorality of individuals. The arguments in this chapter support efforts to move the culture of healthcare organizations away from blaming individuals towards an analysis of systemic sources of error (Department of Health 1999). Although there has been a growing realization that the 'blame culture' which surrounds adverse events in hospital is destructive, there is still a tendency to locate the sources of accidents primarily in the behaviour of individual staff members rather than in the social organization of work.

The focus of sociology is not on the individual but on relationships between or among individuals. Although sociology is a broad church encompassing many different approaches, the focus tends not to be on intra-psychic phenomena or on the individual's subjective experiences, but on the behaviour of individuals in relation to others. Sociology then provides a useful theoretical framework for the study of adverse events because it shifts attention to the group level of analysis.

Organizational sociology has long accepted that mistakes of all kinds are a common, even normal, part of work (Hughes 1951). Indeed, *Normal Accidents* was the title of a book by Charles Perrow (1984) which used standard concepts from organizational theory to explain the nuclear accident at Three Mile Island in the USA and to develop a theory of accident-prone organizations. He argued that to really understand an accident or a failure, we need to start with the individual's mental model of the situation and work outwards towards the organization, industry or government. Perrow (2004) said of *Normal Accidents* that his goal had been to show that 'no matter how hard we might try, certain kinds of systems – those with many non-linear interactions (interactive complexity) and those that are also tightly coupled – were bound to fail eventually'. He distinguished between normal accidents of this type and the more prosaic accidents caused by component failures, within which he included failure of management as well as failures of other equipment. Examples of component failures would be the accidents at Chernobyl and Bhopal, both of which could be traced to management malfeasance.

The aim of this chapter is not to systematically review previous contributions to the sociology of accidents but to illustrate by a few examples how sociological concepts can be used to generate testable hypotheses about the social sources of safety and danger. It aims to strengthen the theoretical basis of future research on adverse events, by drawing on ideas, concepts, and mechanisms from the sociology of organizations where there is a long tradition of studying mistakes, misconduct, and disasters. Until recently this literature has developed in diverse specialties with little cross-fertilization. Experts in disaster research had little contact with researchers focusing on accidents, for example, although they may have relied on many of the same explanatory concepts. This has retarded the development of sociological theory in this area and makes it difficult to generalize from the large number of case studies and anecdotal material that have been generated in the field. This has begun to change. In a comprehensive and judicious review of the literature concerned with organizational deviance, Diane Vaughan (1999) draws out 'theories and concepts that explain, generically, how things go wrong in socially organised settings'. Her review has uncovered causal relationships between the *environment* in which organizations operate, organizational *structures* (including complexity, centralization, and formalization[1]), *processes* (informal organization, power, and learning), and *tasks* (level of skill, technology, and the role of knowledge). The goal of this work was to begin to build the theoretical base for the study of 'the dark side of organizations' as an integrated field. This chapter distils from this review, and from the sociology of organizations more generally, a number of organizational characteristics that can sometimes cast a dark and lingering shadow over patients' experiences in healthcare organizations.

I describe, from a sociological perspective, four intrinsic characteristics of organizations, that are relevant to the level of risk and danger in healthcare settings –

namely, (1) the division of labour in complex organizations; (2) structural holes in communication networks; (3) diffusion of responsibility; and (4) environmental or other pressures that deflect organizations from their main task. I argue that each of these four intrinsic characteristics invokes specific mechanisms that increase danger in healthcare organizations but also offer the possibility of devising strategies and behaviours to increase patient safety. These are not the only organizational features that can affect safety and danger in organizations, but from them a number of testable hypotheses can be derived. If these were tested against empirical data, they would add to the evidence base for developing more effective ways to minimize adverse events in healthcare settings and could contribute to the development of theory in this important area.

The division of labour

We begin with the division of labour – the most fundamental characteristic of organizations – and to some extent their *raison d'être*. The sociological perspective argues that the compartmentalization of work increases the likelihood of adverse events by introducing the need for communication and monitoring. As the number of employees in an organization grows, the number of communication channels increases at an even faster rate. Larger size and increased complexity create greater opportunities for mistakes to occur. Before the Industrial Revolution almost all aspects of social life were based on a few organizations – the church, the manor, and the guild. Those organizations that did exist had a relatively simple structure with little elaboration or differentiation of social roles. Now organizations are not only ubiquitous in social life, they are complex in structure and generate new social roles and positions. Modern health care, scientifically and technologically sophisticated, demands the existence of complex organizations to coordinate the activities of the many individuals required to contribute their specialist expertise.

The division of labour that results from increased specialization brings problems of coordination, communication and cooperation. It is no longer possible for one person to hold all the specialist knowledge needed to treat patients. The members of the healthcare delivery team, who are often educated separately and may have little informal communication (West and Barron (2005)) may have only a limited understanding of each other's role. This is not just because of the increasing scientific and technical sophistication of medical care, but also because of increasing specialization of the occupations and professions involved in health care. The nursing profession, for example, has become increasingly specialized over time and is now recognized as encompassing a large number of groups, each of which is in possession of specialist expertise. Nurses who work in intensive care, psychiatry, or in the community are no longer interchangeable – a 'nurse' is no longer just a 'nurse'. At the same time, the role of the nurse in the healthcare team has become more specialized. Whereas, in the past, nurses were responsible for diverse aspects of patient care, their role is now more clearly defined. Nurses no longer have responsibility for ward cleaning and other ancillary services such as patient transport which could have led to a fragmentation of care and a decline in its quality. The more specialized occupations become, the more room there is for error unless systems for coordination, communication, and cooperation are functioning well. Vaughan (1996) coined the phrase 'structural secrecy' to describe the compart-mentalization of knowledge and information that follows from the division of labour in complex organizations. She identified the following implications of structural secrecy:

- Information and knowledge will always be partial and incomplete.
- The potential for things to go wrong increases when tasks or information cross internal boundaries.
- Segregated knowledge minimizes the ability to detect and stave off activities that deviate from normative standards and expectations.

Structural secrecy emphasizes the importance of communication in formal organiza-tions. If no one individual or group is in possession of full knowledge about the way an organization works or has complete information about its activities, then more emphasis needs to be placed on formal mechanisms of communication. Structural secrecy is one argument for simplifying organizational structures and processes (Berwick 1999).

Standardization and formalization of tasks are ways of reducing the complexity of work in formal organizations. In hospitals, standardization means, for example, that the layout of each ward would be basically the same, procedures would be conducted in the same way across units, and there would be a minimal amount of variation in equipment throughout the organization. Standardization is particularly important if the organization has a high turnover of staff or relies heavily on bank or agency nurses because it minimizes the amount of time wasted on dealing with new or different ways of working. For example, imagine how much easier it would be if all acute wards kept their resuscitation trolleys in exactly the same position and stocked them in exactly the same way. If nurses and doctors do not need to search for the equipment they need, precious time could be saved in an emergency situation. Studying the patterns of accidents and 'near misses' will reveal further ways to simplify and systematize tasks that could be implemented easily and effectively.

Formalization, which refers to the extent to which roles, rules, and procedures are codified and applied within an organization, can also be seen as a way of simplifying tasks because it minimizes the amount of initiative and original thought required of individuals. However, formalization can have negative as well as positive effects. Rules, standard operating procedures, guidelines, protocols, and role specifi-cations cannot cover all eventualities and, unless deliberate steps are taken to review and revise them, they will soon become out of date. Vaughan states: 'recency, per-ceived relevance, complexity, vagueness, and/or acceptability' as factors related to formalization that have been implicated in the past with the systematic production of organizational deviance.

A tendency towards formalization is shown in the growth of the 'guidelines movement' in the healthcare systems of many industrial nations where explicit protocols for treating particularly common diseases such as asthma, diabetes, and back pain have become increasingly visible components of 'evidence-based care'.

Guidelines and protocols are seen as important tools in quality improvement. If, as Vaughan suggests, formalization also carries known dangers, it would seem wise to take these into account. The idea that there are risks associated with increasing formalization is therefore an important caution and suggests that the impact of guidelines and other trends towards formalization should be subject to evaluation and monitoring over time to ensure that the costs do not outweigh the benefits.

The homophily principle and social structural barriers to communication

The homophily principle is the tendency for individuals to form relationships with other people who are like themselves on salient social dimensions, such as education, gender and race (McPherson et al. 2001). Despite the fact that homophily is one of the few ideas in sociology for which there is overwhelming empirical support, it is seldom discussed in medical sociology or in health services research. It is included here because it is an important characteristic of the informal organization of healthcare settings that could also have important ramifications for communication and monitoring.

In healthcare organizations, barriers to communication are erected by the hierarchical nature of hospital organizations, by the importance of professional allegiances, and by the gendered nature of work in healthcare settings. A study of the informal networks of clinical directors and directors of nursing in acute hospitals in the UK National Health Service showed that nurses and doctors rarely discussed important professional matters informally with each other (West and Barron 2005). Most discussion partners were drawn from members of their own professional group, with doctors being most prone to seek out other doctors as discussion partners. Managers were the second most commonly selected discussion partners by both nurses and doctors. Every person in the sample showed a marked preference for discussion partners of their own sex. These findings illustrate how, even in organizations that espouse equal opportunities and that are based on multidisciplinary working, the homophily principle still holds.

Social network analysis has also revealed the tendency, less marked among nurses than among doctors, for professionals' discussion partners to know each other (West et al. 1999). Doctors' social networks were almost like cliques, composed mainly of other doctors, most of whom knew each other and were in frequent, often daily, contact. The density of these social networks suggests that there is still a very strong professional boundary around medicine, which may be very difficult to penetrate. If these findings are generalizable, senior doctors might be described as 'socially insulated' because they have so little contact with people who differ from themselves on important social dimensions such as race, age, income, education, and professional background. When senior doctors and, to a lesser extent, senior nurses discuss important professional matters in informal settings and with discussion partners of their own choosing, they are unlikely to be confronted by ideas or interpretations of the world that differ markedly from their own. At least as far as informal communication goes, there appear to be cliques within hospitals among whom informal communication is frequent but there are also structural barriers based on hierarchy, profession, and sex which make some kinds of relationships unlikely. These boundaries, around medicine in particular, could be a barrier to communication with, and monitoring by, other professional groups.

One of the advantages of an organization promoting safety is the ability to design a system of 'checks and balances' so that important actions are not the sole responsibility of a single individual. For example, powerful drugs are always checked by at least two people before they are administered to the patient. Such organizational arrangements only work, however, if there are few or no social structural barriers to communication between the parties involved. If a junior nurse feels unable to tell her senior partner that she has just drawn up the wrong dose of medication, then the mechanism for ensuring patient safety will break down. Adverse events can happen simply because individuals of lower status experience difficulties in challenging the decision of a person of higher status. Perhaps the most powerful examples of this phenomenon come from flight recorders that reveal the vain attempts of a co-pilot to get the attention of a pilot or to divert them from a course of action that they realize will cause the death of everyone on the flight (McPherson 1998). One sociological study described and analysed the dialogue between pilots, controllers, and cockpit crews in two jumbo jets in fog over Tenerife where the barriers to communication of status, language, and task assignment were contributing factors in a crash in which hundreds of people died (Weick 1991). Further analysis of the dynamics of interprofessional relations using concepts such as status, boundaries, and emotional labour might yield useful insights into the invisible barriers that divide members of a multidisciplinary team.

Diffusion of responsibility

The diffusion of responsibility that can occur in organizations has sometimes been described as 'the problem of many hands' which makes it very difficult to see exactly who is accountable in a long and complex chain of actions. The literature on adverse events and, more generally, on governance in healthcare settings often conveys the impression that determining who is responsible for what in organizations is unproblematic. In fact, it can often be extremely difficult to determine an individual's contribution to patient care, whether good or bad, and this chapter can only begin to suggest some of the ethical implications that ensue from the diffusion of responsibility in healthcare settings.

The problem of 'many hands' means that it can be extraordinarily difficult to discover who is responsible for what in a large organization (Bovens 1998). One philosopher notes that 'With respect to complex organizations, the problem of many hands often turns the quest for responsibility into a quest for the Holy Grail' (Braithwaite 1988). In many cases we simply cannot isolate individual contributions to organizational action. This suggests not only that we lack some of the basic incentives that could be used to increase individual effort in pursuit of quality, but that the ability to achieve justice in organizations is compromised. Some layers of the organizational hierarchy are responsible for decisions that are more visible, concrete, limited in time, and identifiable with specific individuals than are others.

Mistakes are often associated with a particular decision, for example, the decision to prescribe a certain medication, to remove a particular drain, or to decrease the intensity of observation of a psychiatric patient. If these decisions are followed by adverse events, it usually seems that the decision-maker was 'at fault'. Those who are engaged in clinical work are more vulnerable to blame than are people in other positions and at other levels in the healthcare setting. The legal literature has long been aware that people at the top and bottom of organizations tend not to be blamed when accidents happen (Braithwaite 1988). Attention tends to focus on people in the middle – that is, those who are sufficiently senior to make important and visible decisions but insufficiently senior to be cloaked by the diffusion of responsibility that lies over senior managers.

Interviews with clinicians and managers in acute trusts revealed that decision-making patterns in hospitals are similar to other organizations in this respect (West et al. 2000). Whereas at operational levels decisions tended to be highly visible and to have a recognized beginning, middle and end, at higher levels, decisions were much less clear-cut. Doctors working as clinical directors, nurses in ward manager positions, and managers in divisions and directorates were well able to describe the kinds of decisions for which they were primarily responsible but senior managers were not. Senior managers described a decision-making process which was fundamentally 'evolutionary' and consensual, where negotiations continued with many individuals and groups over long periods of time.

The distinction between active and latent failures is important because it captures the temporal and status dimensions associated with different kinds of failures. The work on decision-making draws out these distinctions and emphasizes differences in the processes of decision-making such as visibility and identifiability. In health care we are acutely aware of the behaviour of individual decision-makers (Wilson et al. 1999) but we often fail to follow the causal chain back to the managers, civil servants, or politicians who may have failed in repeated decisions over many years to provide an environment conducive to patient safety.

The environment of organizations

The organizational literature is replete with examples of how organizations set up for one purpose come to strive for other, very different, goals. It seems important to remember that hospitals and other organized healthcare settings are extremely vulnerable to wider socio-economic and political pressures that can divert energy into goals that are not directly related to patient care. The aim of this section is not to make a political point but to draw attention to the fact that the sources of danger to patients are often somewhat removed from the organization itself.

Following the famous study of the Tennessee Valley Authority by Selznick (1949), a stream of research has described how the original goals of an organization can be changed, subverted, or undermined. These changes are often caused by environmental pressures to which the organization has to respond, sometimes in order to survive. The legitimacy of healthcare organizations is at least partly dependent on their espousal of altruistic goals – to care for and, if possible, to cure patients of discomfort, disability, and disease. One of the threats to these goals is the need for organizations to remain economically viable. Financial goals for different healthcare organizations vary depending on the nature of the system to which they belong, as well as over time. The economic pressures on healthcare organizations are probably quite different in the USA and the UK, for example, and we have some empirical evidence that the importance of economic goals has varied over time in the UK.

In qualitative research on clinical effectiveness and clinical management (West 1995, 1996) many participants voiced the opinion that economic goals had assumed too great an importance in the NHS. Some examples include:

> I don't feel that there is a top-down drive for clinical standards. The focus is on things like waiting times. Middle and upper management don't have a clinical background and don't care about standards.
>
> (Clinical Director)

> The public service ethic is still there – it is kept alive by the professions while the organization has been diverted into business activity.
>
> (Academic)

> It's a confused culture at the moment. Dominant requirements of finance and quantitative performance – brute managerialism – but there is a growing recognition that this is demotivating.
>
> (Chief Executive)

Although the current UK government has given clear messages that quality of care takes priority over other goals, at the same time this goal is subverted by the patent inadequacy of funding provided for the NHS. The connection between resources and risk has been established in the literature on high reliability organizations. Among the many characteristics shared by high reliability organizations is the fact that they 'enjoy abundant resources so that short term efficiencies can be neglected in favour of reliable operation' (Sagan 1993). Although such abundance may never be possible in the healthcare context, the difficulties involved in meeting all the current demands on the system when UK spending on health care remains so low in comparison with other countries need to be acknowledged. If top managers set goals that cannot be met with current resources, they are setting up individual clinicians, teams, and organizations for failure of all different kinds, including causing harm to patients.

The implications of this perspective

Sociology can contribute to the development of a more general theoretical approach on which future efforts to decrease risk can be based. The main problem with anecdotal or case study approaches to the analysis of adverse events is that it is all too easy to dismiss any lessons that might be learned by saying 'it couldn't happen here'. Theories assist in the transfer of knowledge from one setting to another so that healthcare professionals can draw on the experiences of such catastrophes as the *Challenger* launch decision (Boisjoly et al. 1996; Vaughan 1996), aeroplane crashes (Weick 1991; McPherson 1998), and chemical and nuclear spills such as occurred at Three Mile Island (Perrow 1981), Prince William Sound (Clarke 1992), Bhopal (Shrivastava

1987) and Chernobyl (Hohenemser 1988). Although these high profile cases may at first seem to have little in common with adverse events in hospitals, they are linked by the fact that organizational structure, process, task and/or environmental pressure are almost always implicated in their production (Vaughan 1999). At the same time, the literature on 'high reliability organizations' is also relevant. Studies of organizations where failures would lead to major disasters, such as aircraft carriers (Roberts 1990) and the US air traffic system (LaPorte 1988), show that organizations that manage to operate reliably and routinely without accidents share a number of features. Scott (1992) lists a number of organizational elements that appear to promote high reliability including 'selection and training of personnel, redundancy of functions (equipment, procedures), reliance on collegiality and negotiation within a tight formal command structure, and a culture emphasising cooperation and commitment to high standards'.

The four areas described above can lead to the generation of a number of testable hypotheses (see Box 2.1) which give direction to future research in this area from a sociological perspective. These ideas are meant to suggest some of the ways in which future research could pursue the sociological approach to the study of adverse events.

Box 2.1 Some testable hypotheses for sociological explanations of the causes of adverse events

- The more easily a named individual can be identified as responsible for co-ordinating the care of a patient, the lower the risk of adverse events.
- The greater the emphasis placed on arrangements for formal communication, the lower the risk of adverse events.
- The more that key tasks such as drug administration, resuscitation, and the prevention of infection are systematized and formalized, the lower the risk of adverse events.
- The more attention given by an organization to celebrating the role of individuals in the promotion of patient safety and high quality care, the lower the risk of adverse events.
- The more responsibility for decreasing the number and seriousness of adverse events is seen as an organizational as well as individual responsibility, the lower the risk of adverse events.
- The greater the number of individuals (departments) involved in the care of a patient, the higher the risk of adverse events.
- The more complex (technologically sophisticated, demanding specialist expertise) the tasks involved in the care of a patient, the higher the risk of adverse events.
- The more that status distinction is observed among professional groups and between men and women in an organization, the higher the risk of adverse events.
- The greater the environmental pressure on an organization to achieve targets that are not directly related to quality of care, the higher the risk of adverse events.
- The more the culture of the organization espouses goals that are not directly related to the quality of patient care, the higher the risk of adverse events.
- The greater the discrepancy between the goals of the organization and the funds available to achieve the goals, the higher the risk of adverse events.

It seems clear that further empirical work on the effect of system simplicity, standardization and formalization – as well as status differences, role boundaries, job design, and environmental pressures – on rates of adverse events would be theoretically justified. Although sociological mechanisms are now widely accepted as implicated in patient safety (Institute of Medicine 1999, 2001), their causal role is, as yet, not well understood. Hoff et al. (2004) conducted a review of the literature examining links between the social organization of heath care, medical errors and patient safety. They concluded that, 'there is little evidence for asserting the importance of any individual, group or structural variable in error prevention or enhanced patient safety at the present time'. They were critical of the existing empirical literature for its lack of a systematic theoretical framework and for its failure to define independent and dependent variables in ways that were theoretically justifiable. Few studies looked at the system level of analysis. Most of the 42 empirical studies included in their review examined the impact of only one independent variable. They attribute some of these deficiencies in the quality of the research in this area to the fact that the field is relatively new. Most of the studies they reviewed had been published since 2000. They are cautious therefore about the extent to which these findings should be implemented in practice. They recommend that managers should do the following:

1. Prioritize the safety issues that the organization needs to address.
2. Specify what outcomes they would like to see for each issue and ensure that accurate data are collected.
3. Implement different interventions and compare their costs and benefits.

Without such an approach, 'the wrong types of organizational dynamics might end up being promoted within the setting over time'. There is a clear need then for more and better quality research in this area to show which, if any, sociological mechanisms affect patient safety. The study of adverse events is extremely important because it combines compassion for patients with concern for healthcare workers, recognizing that these two are inextricably linked. Both groups deserve a better evidence base about how sociology can contribute to the production of a safe and effective healthcare system.

Acknowledgements

This chapter was originally published as a paper entitled 'Organizational sources of safety and danger: sociological contributions to the study of adverse events', in the *Journal of Quality and Safety in Health Care*, 9: 120–6 (2000), and has been substantially revised for this book.

Note

1 Formalization is covered in greater detail in Chapter 16 of this book.

Box 2.2 Key points

- Sociological studies of adverse events focus on levels of analysis above the level of the individual.
- Sociologists have long regarded adverse events as an inevitable, indeed normal, part of work.
- Complex organizations are vulnerable to breakdowns in communication and co-ordination.
- The tendency for individuals to relate to others like themselves creates barriers between groups.
- Identifying who is ultimately responsible for organizational outcomes can be difficult.
- Environmental pressures can deflect organizations from their main goals.
- Empirical evidence linking social organization to adverse events is scarce.
- Testable hypotheses about the social causes of adverse events can be derived from sociological theory and mechanisms.

References

Berwick, D.M. (1999) Improving patient safety: the need and the opportunity, paper presented at the Fourth Annual European Forum on Quality Improvement in Health Care, Stockholm, Sweden.

Boisjoly, R., Curtis, E.F. and Mellican, E. (1996) The *Challenger* disaster: organizational demands and personal ethics, in D.M. Ermann and R.J. Lundman (eds) *Corporate and Governmental Deviance: Problems of Organizational Behaviour in Contemporary Society.* 5th edn. Oxford: Oxford University Press.

Bovens, B. (1998) *The Quest for Responsibility: Accountability and Citizenship in Complex Organizations.* Cambridge: Cambridge University Press.

Braithwaite, J. (1988) The allocation of responsibility for corporate crime: individualism, collectivism and accountability, *Sidney Law Review,* 12: 468–513.

Clarke, L. (1992) The wreck of the *Exxon Valdez,* in D. Nelkin (ed.) *Controversies: Politics of Technical Decisions.* Beverley Hills, CA: Sage, pp. 80–96.

Department of Health (1999) *Clinical Governance: Quality in the New NHS.* London: The Stationery Office.

Hoff, T., Jameson, L., Hannan, E. and Flink, E. (2004) A review of the literature examining linkages between organizational factors, medical errors, and patient safety, *Medical Care Research and Review,* 61(1): 3–37.

Hohenemser, C. (1988) The accident at Chernobyl: health and environmental consequences and the implications for risk management, *Annual Review of Energy and the Environment,* 13: 383–428.

Hughes, E.C. (1951) Mistakes at work, *Canadian Journal of Economic and Political Science,* 17: 320–7.

Institute of Medicine (1999) *To Err Is Human: Building a Safer Health System.* Washington, DC: National Academy Press.

Institute of Medicine (2001) *Crossing the Quality Chasm: A New Health System for the 21st Century.* Washington, DC: National Academy Press.

LaPorte, T.R. (1988) The United States air traffic system: increasing reliability in the midst of rapid growth, in T. Hughes and R. Mayntz (eds) *The Development of Large Scale Technical Systems*. Boulder, CO: Westview Press, pp. 215–44.

Leape, L.L. (1997) A systems analysis approach to medical error, *Journal of Evaluation in Clinical Practice*, 3: 213–22. [*Medline.*]

MacPherson, M. (1998) *The Black Box: Cockpit Voice Recorder Accounts of In-Flight Accidents.* London: HarperCollins.

McPherson, M., Smith-Lovin, L. and Cook, J.M. (2001) Birds of a feather: homophily in social networks, *Annual Review of Sociology*, 27: 415–44.

Perrow, C. (1981) *The Accident at Three Mile Island: The Human Dimension.* Boulder, CO: Westview Press.

Perrow, C. (1984) *Normal Accidents: Living with High-Risk Technologies.* New York: Basic Books.

Perrow, C. (2004) A personal note on *Normal Accidents*, *Organization and Environment*, 17(1): 9–24.

Roberts, K.H. (1990) Some characteristics of one type of high reliability organization, *Organization Science*, 1: 160–76.

Sagan, S.D. (1993) *The Limits of Safety: Organizations, Accidents and Nuclear Weapons.* Princeton, NJ: Princeton University Press.

Scott, W.R. (1992) *Organizations: Rational, Natural and Open Systems.* 3rd edn. Englewood Cliffs, NJ: Prentice Hall.

Selznick, P. (1949) *TVA and the Grass Roots.* Berkeley, CA: University of California Press.

Shrivastava, P. (1987) *Bhopal: Anatomy of a Crisis.* Cambridge, MA: Ballinger.

Vaughan, D. (1996) *The Challenger Launch Decision.* Chicago: Chicago University Press.

Vaughan, D. (1999) The dark side of organizations: mistake, misconduct and disaster, *Annual Review of Sociology*, 25: 271.

Vincent, C. (1997) Risk, safety and the dark side of quality, *British Medical Journal*, 314: 1775–6. [*Free Full Text.*]

Weick, K. (1991) The vulnerable system: an analysis of the Tenerife air disaster, in P. Frost, L. Moore, M. Louis, et al. (eds) *Reframing Organizational Culture.* Newbury Park, CA: Sage, pp. 117–30.

West, E. (1995) *Clinical Effectiveness.* Report prepared for the Clinical Standards Advisory Group. London: Department of Health.

West, E. (1996) *Clinicians in Management.* Report prepared for the Clinical Standards Advisory Group. London: Department of Health.

West, E. and Barron, D.N. (2005) Social and geographical boundaries around the networks of senior nurses and doctors: an application of social network analysis, *Canadian Journal of Nursing Research*, 37–8.

West, E., Barron, D., Dowsett, J., et al. (1999) Hierarchies and cliques in the social networks of health care professionals, *Social Science and Medicine*, 48: 633–46. [*Medline.*]

West, E., Kitson, A., Savage, J., et al. (2000) *Who Decides: Centralization and Decentralization in Acute NHS Trusts.* Final report to NHS R&D Programme on the Organization and Management of Services. London: Department of Health.

Wilson, R.M., Harrison, B.T., Gibberd, R.W., et al. (1999) An analysis of the causes of adverse events from the Quality in Australian Health Care Study, *The Medical Journal of Australia*, 170: 411–15. [*Medline.*]

3
Psychological approaches to patient safety
Dianne Parker and Rebecca Lawton

Psychological approaches

Psychology has produced many insights into the nature and causes of human error. Inspired by the pioneering work of Donald Broadbent, during and after the Second World War, experimental research on human error has been complemented by field research. A great deal of applied research has been prompted by calls from managers in high risk industries for psychologists to help them reduce incidents and accidents, 80 per cent of which are known to be the result of human error (Hale and Glendon 1987). As a result of this research effort, several key distinctions have been made that deepen understanding of human error and its reduction.

The first distinction to be considered contrasts slips/lapses and mistakes. Reason (1990) defined error as 'the failure of planned actions to achieve their desired ends – without the intervention of some unforeseeable event'. In these terms, while a slip represents a problem with the execution of a good plan, a mistake involves an inappropriate or incorrect plan that is correctly executed. Slips and mistakes map directly onto Rasmussen's (Rasmussen and Jensen 1974; Rasmussen 1990) differentiation of three levels of human performance. According to Rasmussen's model, the cognitive mode in which people operate changes as the task performed becomes more familiar, from the knowledge-based through the rule-based to the skill-based level. The three levels are not mutually exclusive, but represent a progression, leading to skilled performance. *Knowledge-based performance*, which involves consciously thinking the task through, is relevant when the task faced is novel and conscious effort must be made to construct a plan of action from stored knowledge. Knowledge-based performance is necessary if, for example, you are planning to drive to a destination never previously visited. Errors at this level of performance are mistakes, arising from incorrect knowledge or from the limitations of cognitive resources. Moreover, decision-making itself is subject to a range of biases (Parker and Lawton 2003). For example, Kahneman and Tversky's (1972) classic laboratory experiments identified the availability bias, referring to the fact that probability judgements (for example, judgements of the likelihood of having a car accident) are strongly influenced by the ease with which past cases can be recalled.[1]

Rule-based performance occurs when we already have some familiarity with the task, and can perform it by drawing on a set of stored mental if–then rules. For example, a learner driver may have learned the appropriate routine for negotiating a roundabout, but will still probably have to give the task full concentration, retrieving the rules and applying them appropriately. Errors at this level are also mistakes, involving the misapplication of a rule, for example, misremembering the correct lane to be taken when turning right at a roundabout. At the *skill-based level of performance* tasks are familiar and actions occur without conscious thought. For example, experienced drivers give little thought to changing gear, steering or using the brakes and are able to combine these tasks with others such as talking to a passenger or monitoring hazards on the road ahead. At this level of performance, errors come in the form of slips and lapses. For example, driving towards work when you intend to go to the supermarket because you are distracted by the children at the point on the route where a different turning is required.

Having established the distinction between slips/lapses and mistakes, a second distinction has been made between these types of error and *violations*. The unifying characteristic of slips, lapses and mistakes is that they are all unintentional. These different types of error all arise from information processing problems, their occurrence can be understood in relation to the cognitive processes of a single individual, and their frequency can be reduced by skills training, improving knowledge, the provision of better information and redesign.

In contrast, violations often have less to do with knowledge or skills and much more to do with motivation. The chief characteristic of a violation is that it represents a deliberate deviation from normal or recommended practice: it is, at least in part, intentional. The frequency of violations cannot usually be reduced by competence assessment or training, because violations reflect what the individual decides to do, rather than what he/she *can* do. In the context of organizational safety, a reduction in violations can best be achieved by attention to aspects of the organization such as morale, attitudes, beliefs, norms and organizational safety culture (Reason et al. 1998).

Violations represent deviations from formal or informal rules that supposedly describe the best/safest way of performing a task, for example, a railwayman who steps on and off a moving shunting engine in order to save time. In this case although the action was intended, the occasionally bad consequences were not. For the most part, violations go unpunished but occasionally and often in combination with an error, the results can be catastrophic. Violations are of particular interest in an organizational context where rules, guidelines, policies and protocols are often developed to control practice (Johnson and Gill 1993) and prevent mistakes (see Chapter 15).

Violations can also be sub-divided into types (Lawton 1998; Reason et al. 1998). Routine violations occur when individuals believe that they have sufficient skill and experience to violate rules habitually, for example, where failure to wear a safety helmet is widespread throughout a workforce. Situational violations occur when the local situation makes following the rules difficult or impossible. Continuing with the safety helmet example, if an insufficient number of safety helmets were provided by management, then failing to wear one would be a situational violation. Optimizing violations serve the needs of the violator to express mastery and skill and may be the province of the very experienced staff member. Some individuals might choose not to wear a safety helmet, perceiving them to be uncomfortable or embarrassing to wear. Finally, the exceptional violation occurs when a novel situation arises which cannot be dealt with in accordance to existing rules. For example, a safety helmet may restrict movement and so become a safety hazard in a confined area. Nevertheless, failure to wear one represents the contravention of a well-known safety rule.

Applying the psychological perspective to the issue of patient safety

With respect to patient safety, there is a growing recognition that an understanding of the nature and frequency of error is a prerequisite for effective error management. However, several researchers have pointed out that achieving a good understanding of failure in health care is hampered by the fact that there is no standard way of defining errors in health care, and therefore no standardized classification system (JCAHO patient safety taxonomy 2003; Sandars and Esmail 2003). Furthermore, there is little uniformity in the way in which events are reported, so that the same event may be given a different classification by different coders (Sutcliffe 2004; Tamuz et al. 2004).

Consequently, researchers have begun to develop taxonomies of medical error. For example, Dovey et al. (2002) used data collected from 42 British GPs on 330 medical errors to develop a preliminary taxonomy of medical error. Their classification distinguishes between errors relating to the process of care, for example, in ordering investigations, managing appointments, completing documentation, treatments and communication and errors relating to knowledge or skills, for example, errors in diagnosis or treatment decisions. This and other taxonomies (including those used in the Harvard RMF, Eindhoven, and National Reporting and Learning Systems system) have in common a bottom-up approach, collecting data about individual errors and clustering them together at coding (see Chapter 7). However, few of the existing taxonomies are derived from a consideration of the psychology of error, which could inform a top-down approach, classifying reported adverse events in terms of the types of error and violation outlined above.

The psychological approach goes beyond description, and moves towards explanation, because it includes a consideration of the cognitive and motivational underpinnings of error. Indeed, Zhang (Zhang et al. 2004) has acknowledged the importance of this approach in health care, suggesting that without a theoretical foundation, '[it] will be difficult to understand the fundamental factors and mechanisms of the problem such that medical errors can be prevented or greatly reduced systematically on a large scale'. Zhang goes on to provide a cognitive taxonomy of medical errors, based on the theoretical model of Reason (1990) and the action theory proposed by Norman (1981). Although Leape (1994) is not explicit about the psychological underpinning, his early classification is based on the distinction between errors and violations and slips and mistakes. Leape divides errors into diagnostic, treatment and preventive errors. Within these categories he also distinguishes between errors that involve omission that is, not doing something one is supposed to and errors of commission, that is, performing an intended action incorrectly or performing an unintended action in the process. Finally, Leape distinguishes between technical errors (the incorrect execution of a correct action) and judgmental (deciding on an inappropriate course of action).

An approach grounded in psychological theory, classifying adverse events in health care according to the distinctions described above, would be of particular benefit to those concerned with the improvement of patient safety. Each of the error and violation types outlined above is easily identifiable in the behaviour of healthcare professionals. For example, consider the situation in which a hospital patient is given the wrong blood in a transfusion. This unfortunate event may have occurred because the nurse concerned failed to read the label on the blood bag properly (an error) or because she did not perform the necessary checks (a violation). Similarly, a patient under anaesthesia may have a cardiac arrest with no warning. This may occur because the annual maintenance check for equipment had been forgotten (an error) or because the anaesthetist, irritated by false alarms, had turned the alarm off (a violation). In both cases, using a conventional classification system would not allow us to distinguish between a true error and a violation.

Considering the sub-types of true errors, it is important to be able to distinguish skill-based, rule-based and knowledge-based errors. In the first example the nurse may have made a skill-based error – she may have been distracted and simply omitted a step in a well-learned sequence of actions. Alternatively, she may have mistakenly thought that the container from which the blood bag was taken was one she had previously identified as containing the patient's blood (a rule-based error). Again, she may have been a relatively inexperienced nurse who simply did not realize that the checking was her responsibility (a knowledge-based error). While the first of these three types of error probably suggest that this nurse would benefit from some redesign of the task environment, to avoid distraction, the third type demands training or re-training in basic procedures.

It is also possible that the nurse omitted the check knowingly, in violation of well-established procedures. It may be the case that the double checking of blood bags is commonly omitted in the Directorate she works in (a routine violation) or, on that particular day, the theatre team were short-staffed, and everyone else was busy at the crucial moment (a situational violation). On the other hand, this may be a very experienced nurse who feels that someone with her level of expertise does not need her actions to be checked, and can save the team a couple of moments by not bothering (an optimizing violation). The appropriate remedy depends crucially on the violation type. The reduction or elimination of routine violations requires a team-, or Directorate-based education programme, while the situational violation described could best be tackled by ensuring adequate staffing levels. While optimizing violations may be performed for laudable reasons, perpetrators should be made aware that the most experienced staff are often those who are involved in the most serious adverse events, when they decide to bend the rules.

Early psychological contributions to an understanding of accidents were based on 'accident proneness', the idea that some individuals have personality characteristics that make them more prone to accidents (cf. Lawton and Parker 1998). This became known as the person-centred approach and focused attention and blame on the individual involved. This is psychologically satisfying, because by blaming someone, particularly if they are dismissed or retrained, we feel the risk of another accident disappears. However, this approach does not do justice to the multi-determined nature of most incidents in complex systems. Once a culpable individual has been found, the investigation tends to be closed, and opportunities for organizational learning may be missed. Moreover, in an organizational culture where individuals attract personal blame for adverse events, the likelihood is that such events will go unreported whenever possible. This means that the organization will never have a clear grasp of the range and nature of the threats to safety it faces.

The systems approach to risk management adopts a more sophisticated perspective, focusing not only on the individual, but also on the role of organizational factors (Reason 2000). It is acknowledged that in order to understand the roots of individual error it is necessary to consider the physical, social and organizational environment in which individuals operate. From the systems perspective, a crucial distinction is made between active and latent failures. Active failures are the proximal causes of adverse events. They nearly always involve individual error or violation and have an immediate negative effect. Latent or organizational failures, on the other hand, are likely to be removed in time and space from the focal event, but nevertheless act as contributory factors. Latent failures, also sometimes known as error-provoking conditions, include poor management, poorly maintained equipment, unworkable procedures or short-sighted policies. These may not lead directly to an adverse event, but make it more likely that one will occur. James Reason's Swiss cheese model, shown in Figure 3.1, offers a widely cited and elegant depiction of the effects of latent failures.

The benefits of the systems approach have been acknowledged in both the USA and the UK, through seminal policy documents: the Institute of Medicine's *To Err Is Human* (1999) and the Department of Health's *Organization with a Memory* (2000). Both reports suggest that one prerequisite for learning from and preventing failures is a clear understanding of the range and number of failures that are occurring in the system. Therefore, one of the key recommendations of both reports was the introduction of a reporting scheme for adverse events and near misses in health care, to provide a database of errors, and allow for the identification of areas of particular

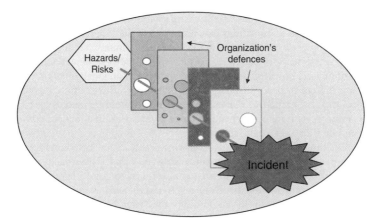

Figure 3.1 The Swiss cheese model of organizational safety
Source: After Reason (1997)

concern. In England, one of the primary functions of the National Patient Safety Agency (NPSA) was the development of a reporting system, the National Reporting and Learning System (NRLS).

Investigating the psychological origins of the behaviour that gave rise to an adverse event can help investigators decide on the most appropriate action to take in order to prevent such an event occurring again. However, it can also elucidate the latent failures that have contributed to the error or violation in the first place. Research on error types in a range of high-risk industries has identified factors such as teamwork, communications, design and training to have an impact of error rates (Helmreich 2000; Mearns et al. 2001). Many of these factors would not be readily identified by an approach that focused narrowly on what happened, rather than why. Investigatory techniques such as root cause analysis are very valuable in uncovering the latent failures that underlie active failures in a complex adverse event. However, it is also important to understand the psychological aetiology of both active and latent failures, that is, whether each failure identified was an error or a violation.

The advantages and disadvantages of psychological approaches to patient safety

The practical usefulness of the error–violation distinction lies in the fact that it highlights the need for different remedies in trying to improve patient safety. The incidence of true error can be minimized through the use of defences as described in Reason's Swiss cheese model. However, the commission of violations in an organization arises from the attitudes and values of the members of that organization. In other words, the tendency for violations to occur is a reflection of the culture of the organization. In terms of patient safety, organizational safety culture manifests itself through aspects of the organization such as the way in which adverse events are investigated, through communication about safety, team working on safety and education and training on safety (see Chapter 14 for a detailed description of a framework for understanding organizational safety culture in health care). These are precisely the kind of factors that have been identified in other high-risk industries as crucial for the safety health of organizations. Violations are likely to flourish where there are only superficial attempts to report and investigate incidents, where there is a culture of poor communication or poor safety training and education. It is apparent from recent reviews (e.g., Flin et al. 2000) that core aspects of organizational safety culture include work pressure, competence, and management/supervision. Unreasonable work pressure will make both error and violation more likely, while inadequate competency assessment will lead to errors from insufficiently skilled staff, and poor management and/or supervision is likely to allow, or even encourage, the commission of violations.

There is growing evidence that utilizing the psychological approach can facilitate organizational learning. Two recent, high profile inquiries into serious adverse incidents in the UK, Bristol Royal Infirmary (Kennedy 2001) and Queens Medical Centre (Toft 2001) have adopted the systems approach and, in doing so, have highlighted serious problems in the management of safety in the NHS. These problems include inadequate systems for reporting, a consistent failure within organizations to learn from mistakes, and organizational cultures that focus on blame rather than safety. At the same time, these reports have been useful models for organizational learning. For example, the proximal cause of the fatal intrathecal injection of vincristine at Queens Medical Centre (QMC) was shown to arise from a combination of errors and violations. However, a wide range of situational and organizational factors that had contributed to the incident were also identified in the report, including labelling of syringes, problems with communication between staff, conflicting protocols and the design of medical devices. Moreover, there is a growing recognition internationally that in developing strategies to improve patient safety, a systems approach is essential. For example, a recent Institute of Medicine, US publication (Page 2004) documents the role of the work environment of nurses in keeping patients safe. In a separate document published by The Change Foundation, Canada (Wong and Beglaryan 2004), strategies for improving patient safety include areas such as leadership, culture, training and reporting.

Other recent research has also investigated the situational and organizational factors implicated in adverse event reports. For example, Dean, Schachter, Vincent and Barber (2002) interviewed healthcare professionals involved in 44 prescribing errors. They identified that the majority of the errors were the result of attentional slips or rule violations. They also elicited information about the organizational factors that had a role in causing these errors. Work environment, workload, team communication were all identified as contributory factors. In another study involving interviews with eight members of staff to systematically analyse a serious incident on an acute psychiatric ward (Vincent et al. 2000), organizational problems such as deficiencies in training and supervision and poor communication emerged as likely causal factors.

Incident investigations that take into account the error–violation distinction, and the need to establish distal as well as proximal causes, are more likely to lead to organizational learning in the NHS. However, such learning predominantly occurs as a reaction to an adverse patient safety incident. In other high-risk industries this reactive approach is complemented by a more proactive error management strategy (Vincent 2001). Proactive organizational learning involves the measurement of the organization's safety health (Reason 1997). For example, teamwork, communication, procedures, protocols, staffing and equipment availability might be identified as factors that correlate with the likelihood of error. By monitoring these factors, through staff and patient surveys, managers can access information on which areas to focus attention and resources in order to reduce errors. A useful metaphor that helps clarify this distinction between the reactive and proactive approaches (Reason, personal communication) is the case of malaria. The risk of malaria can be reduced by swatting each mosquito that you see. However, a more effective way of reducing malaria is to identify where the mosquitoes are coming from before they do harm, that is, drain the swamps in which the mosquitoes breed. Thus, reactive approaches tend to tackle the errors one-by-one, whereas proactive approaches address the organizational factors before they give rise to error.

While attempting to manage error proactively seems an intuitively sensible approach, there is currently very little reliable empirical research investigating the efficacy of organizational level interventions in reducing error in health care. This is partly because many studies are not well designed and reported. Hoff et al.'s (2004) review of 42 healthcare research studies identified only seven properly controlled experimental studies. Even more disappointingly, 80 per cent of the studies provided insufficient detail of the method or findings to allow the strength of the relationship between organizational factors and error to be determined. Most disappointing was the fact that only 38 per cent of the studies reviewed were underpinned by a theoretical framework.

To conclude, the drive towards improving patient safety and reducing medical error is gaining momentum. To avoid reinvention of the wheel, researchers and safety practitioners in health care should take advantage of what has already been learned by psychologists, both in the experimental laboratory and in other high-risk industries. The psychological literature on human error has elucidated several important distinctions in terms of error types, and appropriate remediation strategies. In this chapter we have tried to show how a consideration of those distinctions can be helpful when applied in the context of health care.

Note

1   For more on how these biases influence medical decision-making, see Bogardus et al. (1999).

Box 3.1 Key points

- Psychology has made an important contribution to improving safety in a range of high-risk industries.
- Patient safety practitioners and researchers could benefit from what has already been learned in other industries.
- The systems approach to patient safety allows for the identification of latent organizational failures as well as active individual failures.
- The most useful taxonomies of error, for those seeking to improve patient safety are those based on human error theory, that distinguish between unintentional errors and intentional violations.
- Errors and violations demand different types of remedies.
- Utilizing the psychological approach to patient safety facilitates organizational learning.

References

Bogardus, S., Holmboe, E. and Jekel, J. (1999) Perils, pitfalls and possibilities in talking about medical risk, *Journal of the American Medical Association*, 281: 1037–41.

Dean, B., Schachter, M., Vincent, C. and Barber, N. (2002) Causes of prescribing errors in hospital inpatients: a prospective study, *Lancet*, 359: 1373–8.

Department of Health (2000) *An Organization with a Memory*. London: The Stationery Office.

Dovey, S.M., Meyers, D.S., Phillips Jr, R.L., Green, L.A., Fryer, G.E., Galliher, J.M., Kappus, J. and Grob, P. (2002) A preliminary taxonomy of medical errors in family practice, *Quality and Safety in Health Care*, 11: 233–8.

Flin, R., Mearns, K., O'Connor, P. and Bryden, R. (2000) Measuring safety climate: identifying the common features, *Safety Science*, 34: 177–92.

Hale, A.R. and Glendon, A. (1987) *Individual Behaviour in the Control of Danger*. New York: Elsevier Science.

Helmreich, R.L. (2000) On error management: lessons from aviation, *British Medical Journal*, 320: 781–5.

Hoff, T., Jameson, L., Hannan, E. and Flink, E. (2004) A review of the literature examining linkages between organizational factors, medical errors and patient safety, *Medical Care Research and Review*, 61: 3–37.

Institute of Medicine (1999) *To Err Is Human: Building a Safer Health System*. Washington, DC: National Academy Press.

Johnson, P. and Gill, J. (1993) *Management Control and Organizational Behaviour*. London: Paul Chapman.

Kahneman, D. and Tversky, A. (1972) Subjective probability: a judgement of representativeness, *Cognitive Psychology*, 3(3): 430–54.

Kennedy, I. (2001) *Learning from Bristol: The Report of the Public Inquiry into Children's Heart Surgery at the Bristol Royal Infirmary 1984–1995*. CM 5207. London: The Stationery Office.

Lawton, R. (1998) Not working to rule: understanding procedural violations at work, *Safety Science*, 28: 77–95.

Lawton, R.L. and Parker, D. (1998) Individual differences in accident liability: a review and integrative approach, *Human Factors*, 40: 655–71.

Leape, L.L. (1994) Error in medicine, *Journal of the American Medical Association*, 272: 1851–7.

Mearns, K., Flin, R. and O'Connor, P. (2001) Sharing 'worlds of risk': improving communication with crew resource management, *Journal of Risk Research*, 4(4): 377–92.

Norman, D.A. (1981) Categorization of action slips, *Psychological Review*, 88: 1–15.

Page, A. (2004) *Keeping Patients Safe: Transforming the Work Environment of Nurses*. Washington, DC: National Academy Press.

Parker, D. and Lawton, R. (2003) Psychological contribution to the understanding of adverse events in health care, *Quality and Safety in Health Care*, 12(6): 453–7.

Rasmussen, J. (1990) Human error and the problem of causality in analysis of accidents, *Philosophical Transactions of the Royal Society of London, Series B, Biological Sciences*, 327: 449–60.

Rasmussen, J. and Jensen, A. (1974) Mental procedures in real-life tasks: a case study of electronic troubleshooting, *Ergonomics*, 17: 293–307.

Reason, J. (1990) *Human Error*. Cambridge: Cambridge University Press.

Reason, J. (1997) *Managing the Risks of Organizational Accidents*. Aldershot: Ashgate.

Reason, J. (2000) Human error: models and management, *British Medical Journal*, 320: 768–70.

Reason, J., Parker, D. and Lawton, R. (1998) The varieties of rule-related behaviour, *Journal of Organizational and Occupational Psychology*, 71: 289–304.

Sandars, J. and Esmail, A. (2003) The frequency and nature of medical error in primary care: understanding the diversity across studies, *Family Practice*, 20: 231–6.

Sutcliffe, K.M. (2004) Defining and classifying medical error: lessons for learning, *Quality and Safety in Healthcare*, 13: 8–9.

Tamuz, M., Thomas, E.J. and Franchois, K.E. (2004) Defining and classifying medical error: lessons for patient safety reporting systems, *Quality and Safety in Healthcare*, 13: 13–20.

Toft, B. External inquiry into the adverse incident that occurred at Queen's Medical Centre, Nottingham, 4 January 2001. Available at: www.doh.gov.uk/qmcinquiry/index.htm

Tversky, A. and Kahneman, D. (1974) Judgements under uncertainty, *Science*, 185: 1124–31.
Vincent, C.A. (ed.) (2001) *Clinical Risk Management: Enhancing Patient Safety*. London: BMJ Publications.
Vincent, C., Stanhope, N. and Taylor-Adams, S. (2000) Developing a systematic method of analyzing serious accidents in mental health, *Journal of Mental Health*, 9: 89–103.
Wong, J. and Beglaryan, H. (2004) Strategies for Hospitals to Improve Patient Safety: A Review of Research. The Change Foundation. Available at: www.changefoundation.com.
Zhang, J., Patel, V.L., Johnson, T.R. and Shortliffe, E.H. (2004) A cognitive taxonomy of medical errors, *Journal of Biomedical Informatics*, 37: 193–204.

4

The contribution of quality management to patient safety

Ruth Boaden

What has quality got to do with patient safety – everything or nothing? The two terms appear to be used somewhat interchangeably in the literature and any differences can be argued to be 'a matter of semantics' (Moss and Barach 2002). However, the discipline of quality improvement has a long history, not only in health care, but in other industries where many maintain it has its roots. The field of quality management has a lot to offer the study of patient safety, and this chapter seeks to highlight the key areas where learning could take place. As with the development of any new field of study, there is always a danger of 'reinventing the wheel' and it is argued here that this could be avoided in the study of patient safety if a greater understanding of quality improvement in general could be developed.

The chapter begins with a review of how quality is conceptualized both in general, and within health care specifically, and its relationship to safety. An account of the development of key quality improvement approaches and tools is then given to illustrate the roots of approaches now used within patient safety, focusing on

1. Tools and approaches.
2. Whole systems thinking.
3. The role of people and culture.

The chapter concludes with lessons learned from the quality improvement movement in these areas which may be applicable to the study and improvement of patient safety.

The concept of quality

Quality management/improvement in general (rather than that in health care) can be argued to have developed from the field of production/operations management, which is characterized by an empirical focus. However, the concept of 'quality' is much older, with its formalization sometimes being attributed to the work of Shewhart on statistical process control (SPC) in the 1930s (Shewhart 1931). The term 'quality' is appealing as 'it can be used to legitimize all sorts of measures and changes in the name of a self-evident good' (Wilkinson and Willmott 1995) and definitions of quality abound (Reeves and Bednar 1994). As the study of 'quality' as a concept, and the management of quality within organizations, has developed, a number of fields of study have made contributions – including services marketing, organization studies, human resource management and organizational behaviour, especially change management, much as the field of patient safety now appears to be doing (see Introduction). However, the diverse meanings of the term make it both a 'seductive and slippery philosophy of management' but also 'an elusive topic of study' (Wilkinson and Willmott 1995).

The development of healthcare quality can be argued to have started with the basis of the profession of medicine as a craft developed by Hippocrates (Merry and Crago 2001), with quality based almost solely on the skill of the 'craftspeople' (Reeves and Bednar 1994), and as the concept has been formalized within the healthcare field, a suite of healthcare-related definitions and 'dimensions of quality' have developed (see Table 4.1). A recent development has been the promotion of 'improvement science' as a discipline (Clarke et al. 2004) but its definition and the relationship between this and the more established field of quality management are currently unclear (Boaden et al. 2005). However, the philosophies that underpin quality management and the techniques that are associated with it are increasingly being applied in the healthcare sector in both the USA and Europe. This chapter cannot provide an overview of quality in health care, and this has been done far more thoroughly by e.g. Committee on Quality Health Care in America and Institute of Medicine (2001), while research issues are well covered in Grol et al. (2004).

Until the 1980s most of the emphasis on quality improvement, and most of the empirical utilization of the associated techniques, were within manufacturing industry. However, the field of 'service quality' developed with input from academics from marketing – led from Scandanavia (Groonroos 1984) and the USA (Berry et al. 1985). Many of the quality improvement techniques used in health care have, however, been translated from those used in manufacturing, rather than services, with little attention to date being paid explicitly to the 'service' aspects of healthcare quality.

Quality and safety

The link between quality and safety (if there is one) needs to be clear, as does the issue of whether such a link really matters. Most would agree that 'care cannot be considered to be of high quality unless it is safe' (Moss and Barach 2002), and many of the topics in patient safety journals or papers; teamwork, human factors, leadership, experiential learning, organizational behaviour, change (Moss and Barach 2002), are relevant to all aspects of quality improvement – including safety. Vincent (1997) termed safety the 'dark side of quality' in that the positive dimensions of quality, as described by e.g. Maxwell (1984) may have directed attention away from safety. More recent definitions of quality (see Table 4.1) include 'safety' as one of its key dimensions, and argue that it is a prerequisite for quality: 'achieving a high level of safety is an essential first step in improving the quality of care overall' (Committee on Quality Health Care in America et al. 2001).

Table 4.1 Definitions of healthcare quality

Donabedian (Donabedian 1987)	Maxwell (Maxwell 1984)	Langley et al. (Langley et al. 1996)	Institute of Medicine (Committee on Quality Health Care in America et al. 2001)
Manner in which practitioner manages the personal interaction with the patient	Access to services	Performance	Safety
Patient's own contribution to care	Relevance to need	Features	Effectiveness
Amenities of the settings where care is provided	Effectiveness	Time	Patient-centredness
Facility in access to care	Equity	Reliability	Timeliness
Social distribution of access	Social acceptability, efficiency and economy	Durability	Efficiency
Social distribution of health improvements attributable to care		Uniformity	Equity
		Consistency	
		Serviceability	
		Aesthetics	
		Personal interaction	
		Flexibility	
		Harmlessness	
		Perceived quality	
		Usability	

A review of patient safety research, which included interviews with key funders in the USA (Cooper et al. 2001), concluded that there is 'substantial ambiguity in the definition of patient safety . . . the boundary between safety and quality of care is indistinct', although it argued that the implications are mainly around clarity of funding focus for both funders and applicants, rather than hindering the progress of research *per se*. While most interviewees viewed safety as part of quality, they recognized that there was a tendency to utilize the most fashionable term: 'patient safety has become the issue "du jour" and so almost everything gets redefined in that'.

Tools and approaches

The tools and techniques used for quality improvement in manufacturing, and later in service industries, were developed by a series of individuals (often referred to as 'gurus') from both the USA and Japan following the Second World War (Dale 2003). Details of quality improvement tools from Dale (2003) are presented in Table 4.2. Many of these tools are now used as part of a patient safety approach. The 'golden thread' through all the approaches promoted by these individuals is adopting quality as a fundamental business strategy permeating the culture of the whole organization (McBryde 1986), although most of them are actually remembered for individual tools and techniques which they developed e.g. the Plan-Do-Check-Action (PDCA) cycle, statistical process control (SPC), etc.

Some authors argue that while some of the 'gurus' were working in Japan to pursue 'unending improvement and innovation through mobilising the entire workforce in pursuit of these aims', the West was focusing on 'conformance to standards, control of processes and command of personnel' (Wright 1997) using individual improvement tools, rather than taking an overall holistic approach to improvement, and may still be doing so (Seddon 2003). The main themes of the various individual approaches were summarized by Bendell et al. (1995); these are detailed and referenced in Table 4.3, along with the implications of their various approaches for patient safety. Nielsen et al. (2004) asked the question 'Can the gurus' concepts cure healthcare?' and although the focus was on the overall philosophy rather than the use of individual tools, the analysis does yield some interesting insights. It concluded that Crosby would continue to emphasize the role of leadership in pursuing zero defects, and that Deming would continue to emphasize transformation (as he did in the 14th of his 14 points (Deming 1986)) while being disappointed at the reactive behaviour of healthcare organizations and individuals with 'far too little pursuit of constant improvement' (Nielsen et al. 2004). Feigenbaum's concepts would focus on clearer identification of the customer and the application of evidence-based medicine. Juran's emphasis would be on building quality into processes from the start (what he termed 'quality planning').

Making quality 'total' – whole systems thinking

It has already been shown that many of the quality 'gurus' did not in fact promote single 'tools' for improvement but an overall company-wide approach, although many did not use the term 'total', and the advent of the TQM 'movement' was based on

Table 4.2 Quality improvement tools and techniques and their application in patient safety

Tool	Description	Source (where one identifiable) and application in patient safety
Benchmarking	Learning from the experience of others by comparing products or processes – can be internal (within a company), competitive (with competitors), functional/generic (comparing processes with 'best in class')	Developed from the work at Rank Xerox in the 1980s, documented by Camp (1989)
Brainstorming	Used with a variety of tools to generate ideas in groups	Recommended as a tool for data analysis in NPSA (National Patient Safety Agency 2004) Step 6 – learn and share safety lessons, along with brainwriting
Checklists	Lists of key features of a process, equipment, etc. to be checked	Used in NPSA (National Patient Safety Agency 2004) Step 2 – Lead and support your staff Safety checklist for patient safety leads: 'a range of choices to consider, periodically revisit and use to trigger action' And in Step 3 – Integrate your risk management activity (risk checklist) Also used as Checklist for Assessing Institutional Resilience: tool designed to help health care organizations assess the climate of patient safety in their workplaces (Reason and Wreathall 2005)
Departmental purpose analysis	Tool used to facilitate internal customer relationships	Originated at IBM in 1984
Design of experiments (DOE)	A series of techniques which identify and control parameters which have a potential impact on performance, aiming to make the performance of the system immune to variation	Dates back to agricultural research by Sir R A Fisher in the 1920s, later developed by Taguchi (Taguchi 1986) and adopted in both Japan and the West.

Continued overleaf

Table 4.2 *(Continued)*

Tool	Description	Source (where one identifiable) and application in patient safety
Failure mode and effects analysis (FMEA)	A planning tool used to 'build quality in' to a product or service, for either design or process. It looks at the ways in which the product or service might fail, and then modifies the design or process to avoid these or minimize them.	Developed in 1962 in the aerospace and defence industry as a means of reliability analysis, risk analysis and management. Used in NPSA (National Patient Safety Agency 2004) Step 3 – Integrate your risk management activity Termed 'Failure Mode Effect and Criticality Analysis' (FMECA) by (Joint Commission on Accreditation of Healthcare Organizations 2005) Described by Apkon et al. (2004)
Flowcharts	A basis for the application of many other tools. A diagrammatic representation of the steps in a process, often using standard symbols. Many variations available.	Developed from industrial engineering methods but no one identifiable source. Widely used in systems analysis and business process reengineering.
Housekeeping	Essentially about cleanliness, etc. in the production environment	Based on what the Japanese refer to as the 5s: –*Seiri* – organization –*Seiton* – neatness –*Seiso* – cleaning –*Seiketsu* – standardization –*Shitsuke* – discipline
Mistake-proofing	Technique used to prevent errors turning into defects in the final product – based on the assumption that mistakes will occur, however 'careful' individuals are, unless preventative measures are put in place. Statistical methods accept defects as inevitable, but the source of the mistake should be identified and prevented.	Developed by Shingo (Shingo 1986)

Plan-Do-Check-Act (PDCA) cycle	Developed originally by Deming (Deming 1986)	The basis for the Model for Improvement (Langley et al. 1996) although it is not clear how PDCA became used as Plan-Do-Study-Act (PDSA)
Policy deployment	The western tradition of 'hoshin kanri' – Japanese 'strategic planning and management process involving setting direction and deploying the means of achieving that direction' (Dale 2003). Used to communicate policy, goals and objectives through the hierarchy of the organization, focusing on the key activities for success.	Developed in Japan in early 1960s, concept conceived by Bridgestone Tire Company, and adopted in the US from the early 1980s, with great popularity in large multinationals with Japanese subsidiaries.
Quality costing	Tools used to identify the costs of quality, often using the prevention-appraisal-failure (PAF) categorization	PAF developed by Feigenbaum (Feigenbaum 1961). Cost of (non) conformance developed by Crosby (Crosby 1979)
Quality function deployment	Tool to incorporate knowledge about needs of customers into all stages of design and manufacture/delivery process. Initially translates customer needs into design requirements, based on the concept of the 'Voice of the Customer'. Closely related to FMEA and DOE.	Developed in Japan at Kobe Shipyard
Statistical process control (SPC)	Shewhart (Shewhart 1931) sought to identify the difference between 'natural' variation – termed 'common cause' – and that which could be controlled – 'special' or 'assignable' cause variation. Processes that exhibited only common cause variation were said to be in statistical control. One of the many significant features of this work, which is still used in basically the same form today, is that 'the management of quality acquired a scientific and statistical foundation' (Kolesar 1993). It is regarded as a tool for measurement (Plsek 1999) – 'management control of the process through the use of statistical methods' (Dale 2003)	Roots of SPC can be traced to work in the 1920s in Bell Laboratories (Shewhart 1931)

Continued overleaf

Table 4.2 *(Continued)*

Tool	Description	Source *(where one identifiable) and application in patient safety*
Total productive maintenance	Can be considered as a method of management, combining principles of Productive Maintenance (PM) with TQM.	Developed by the Japanese from the planned approach to PM
The seven quality control tools:		
1. Cause-and-effect diagram	Diagram used to determine and break down the main causes of a given problem – sometimes called 'fishbone' diagrams. Used where there is one problem and the causes may be hierarchical in nature. Can be used by teams or individuals	Ishikawa (Ishikawa 1979) Used as the basis for the Root Cause Analysis process in NPSA (National Patient Safety Agency 2004) Step 6 – learn and share safety lessons 'A retrospective review of a patient safety incident undertaken in order to identify what, how, and why it happened. The analysis is then used to identify areas for change, recommendations and sustainable solutions, to help minimise the re-occurrence of the incident type in the future . . . a methodology that enables you to ask the following questions: What? How? Why?' (National Patient Safety Agency 2004) Described by Senders (2004).
2. Checksheet	Sheet or form used to collect data	Can be similar to a checklist
3. Control chart	The way in which SPC data is displayed, viewed as helping to decide how to improve – whether to search for special causes (if the process is out of control) or work on more fundamental process redesign (if the process is in control). Charts can also be use to monitor improvements over time (Benneyan et al. 2003).	Control charts were used as the basis for SPC development but it is not clear exactly when they were first used.

4. Graphs	Any form of pictorial representation of data	Basic mathematical technique
5. Histogram	Developed from tally charts, basic statistical tool to describe the distribution of a series of data points	Basic mathematical technique
6. Pareto diagram	Technique for prioritizing issues – a form of bar chart with a cumulative percentage curve overlaid on it. Sometimes referred to as the 80/20 rule.	Named after nineteenth-century Italian economist who observed that a large proportion of a country's wealth is held by a small proportion of the population.
7. Scatter diagram	Used to examine the possible relationship between two variables	Basic mathematical technique
The seven management tools (M7):	Generally used in design or sales/marketing areas, where quantitative data is less easy to obtain.	Developed by the Japanese to collect and analyse qualitative and verbal data. Many have already been used in other TQM applications.
1. Affinity diagrams	Used to categorize verbal data/language about previously unexplored vague issues	
2. Arrow diagrams	Applies systematic thinking to the planning and execution of a set of complex tasks	Used in project management as part of critical path analysis (CPA) and programme evaluation and review technique (PERT)
3. Decision programme chart	Used to select the best process to obtain the desired outcome by listing all possible events, contingencies and outcomes	Used in NPSA (National Patient Safety Agency 2004) Step 1 – build a safety culture: Incident Decision Tree: 'created to provide a framework for human resource and NHS managers determining the course of action to take with staff who have been involved in a patient safety incident . . . Based on a model developed by Prof James Reason for the aviation industry, prompts the user with a series of questions to help them take a more systematic, transparent and fair approach to decision-making.' (National Patient Safety Agency 2004) Also similar to Decision Tree for Unsafe Acts Culpability, based on decision trees presented in Reason (1997)

Table 4.2 (Continued)

Tool	Description	Source (where one identifiable) and application in patient safety
4. Matrix data analysis, process	Multivariate mathematical methods used to analyse the data from a matrix diagram	
5. Matrix diagrams	Used to clarify the relationship between results and causes or objectives and methods, using codes to illustrate the direction and relative importance of the influence	Used in NPSA (National Patient Safety Agency 2004) Step 3 – Integrate your risk management activity (along with a model of probabilistic risk assessment)
6. Relations diagrams	Used to identify complex cause-and-effect relationships, where the causes are non-hierarchical and the 'effect' is complex	Some parallels with the use of 'triggers' or clues, to identify adverse events, which is viewed as an effective method for measuring the overall level of harm in a health care organization (Resar et al. 2003) and is first attributed to Jick (1974)
7. Systematic diagrams	Sometimes called a 'tree' diagram – used to examine the most effective means of planning to accomplish a task or solve a problem	– Nominal group technique – Five whys
These tools have no direct parallel with standard quality management tools		Also recommended as data analysis tools in NPSA (National Patient Safety Agency 2004) Step 6 – learn and share safety lessons – Safety climate survey (Sexton et al. 2005) – The SBAR (Situation-Background-Assessment-Recommendation) technique; a framework for communication between members of the health care team (Kaiser Permanente 2005)

Table 4.3 Quality 'gurus': Deming, Juran, Feigenbaum, Ishikawa

'Guru'	Key points of approach	Key points as summarized by Bendell et al. (1995) and references	Patient safety interprets this as . . .
All of them	All the 'gurus' recommend certain tools and techniques, based on the underlying assumption that all work can be described as a process (Boaden et al. 2005)	Tools and techniques are needed (e.g. seven quality control tools promoted by Ishikawa)	Many of the tools promoted by the quality 'gurus' are now promoted as being applicable to the analysis of patient safety incidents (see Table 4.2)
Deming	Influenced by Shewhart (Shewhart 1931) and he developed a 14-point approach for his management philosophy which claimed to improve quality and change organizational culture and has undoubtedly been influential in challenging leaders to 'transform the organization around the concept of continuous improvement' (Vinzant and Vinzant 1999). Responsible for developing the concept of the PDCA (plan–do–check–action) cycle Work started with a focus on a small number of 'tools' for analysis, but developed to a broader methodology which recognized that 'There is no substitute for knowledge' – methods and tools were useful but they did not substitute for this knowledge He called this the 'system of profound knowledge':[1] appreciation for a system, understanding of variation, psychology, and the use of measurement and testing to develop knowledge.	Management commitment and employee awareness are essential Customer focus is key (Deming 1986)	Leadership emphasized in the NPSA Seven Steps to Patient Safety (National Patient Safety Agency 2004), Step 2 and through the various exhortations to develop a safety culture (see Chapter 14) The main customer being the patient – hence the widespread use of the term 'patient safety'. The application of other quality improvement techniques to healthcare is less clear about the patient being the customer because a wide range of stakeholders are identified. If the internal customer-supplier concept which is important in quality improvement is utilized, then the next step in the process is the 'customer' rather than the 'end-user' (which might be interpreted as the patient).

Table 4.3 (Continued)

'Guru'	Key points of approach	Key points as summarized by Bendell et al. (1995) and references	Patient safety interprets this as . . .
Juran	Focused on the managerial aspects of implementing quality Quality, through a reduction in statistical variation, improved productivity and competitive position Quality promoted a trilogy of quality planning, quality control and quality improvement.	Actions need to be planned and prioritized (Juran 1951)	Implicit in most patient safety literature – it refers to effective programme and project management, which is not explicit although clearly necessary. This also refers to the design of processes, something which is again not given very much attention in patient safety at present although this may be changing.
Feigenbaum	Defined quality as a way of managing (rather than a series of technical projects) and the responsibility of everyone. Major contribution was the categorization of quality costs into three: appraisal, prevention and failure Believed that cost reduction was a result of total quality control. Insisted that management and leadership are essential for quality improvement The first to use the term 'total' in relation to quality management Work being described as relevant to health care (Berwick 1989).	Management tools/approaches will be needed as well as detailed quality improvement tools (Feigenbaum 1961)	Some of the tools included in the previous step could be classed as management tools, although the ones used in patient safety to date have been primarily quantitative in nature.
Ishikawa	Contributed thinking on the seven basic quality control tools (Table 4.2), the company-wide quality movement and quality circles, Underlying theme of his work was that 'people at all levels of the organization should use simple methods and work together to solve problems' (Dale 2003)	Teamwork plays a vital part (Ishikawa 1979)	Implicit in the UK (National Patient Safety Agency 2004) Seven Steps document although it can be argued to be an explicit part of healthcare organization working in any case (see Chapter 16)

1 http://www.deming.org/

very similar principles to those which had been promoted for a number of years by these individuals. Quality improvement as an overall approach was developed in the West during the 1980s, following more concerted focus on quality assurance rather than simply quality control (Dale 2003) with the predictable confusion of terminology (Larson and Muller 2002/3): terms used to describe quality improvement include Total Quality Management (TQM), Continuous Quality Improvement (CQI) (McLaughlin and Simpson 1999) and Total Quality Improvement (TQI) (Iles and Sutherland 2001), and such terms appear to be interchangeable in usage. Such an overall approach has been promoted as a 'management philosophy and business strategy' (Hackman and Wageman 1995), although the same authors argue that '[TQM] has become mainly a banner under which a potpourri of essentially unrelated organizational changes are undertaken', and its attractiveness may have been its apparent simplicity; it offers 'a unified set of principles which can guide managers through the numerous choices [open to them] or might even make choosing unnecessary' (Huczynski 1993). Similar claims have been made for other packages of improvement such as Business Process Reengineering (BPR) (McNulty and Ferlie 2002). TQM is based on the following change principles (Hackman and Wageman 1995):

- Focus on work processes.
- Analyse variability.
- Manage by 'fact', i.e. systematically collected data.
- Learning and continuous improvement.

Many of these themes are common with those of the quality 'gurus' with the difference in a TQM approach being the way in which they are 'packaged' as a whole, and the 'all or nothing' way in which it was promoted. The commonest interventions (or 'tools') designed to realize the values of TQM are, according to Hackman and Wageman (1995):

- Explicit identification and measurement of customer requirements.
- Creation of supplier partnerships.
- Use of cross-functional teams to identify and solve quality problems.
- Use of scientific methods to monitor performance and identify areas for performance improvement.
- Use process management approaches to enhance team effectiveness.

Quality improvement in health care as an overall approach (whether or not it has the TQM label) is embodied in the work of the Institute for Healthcare Improvement (IHI), established in 1991 and described as

> 'a not-for-profit organization driving the improvement of health by advancing the quality and value of health care . . . The Institute helps accelerate change in health

care by cultivating promising concepts for improving patient care and turning those ideas into action.'[1]

One of its themes is patient safety and it links this clearly back to some of the broader approaches it recommends for quality improvement, in particular, the model for improvement (Langley et al. 1996). It is notable that IHI is now one of the leaders in the patient safety movement in the USA, and could be said to be adept at packaging the latest 'fad' (Carson et al. 1999) in a way that makes it immediately applicable for healthcare organizations.

The relationship of this development of thinking about quality to a whole systems 'total' view is paralleled in the development of patient safety from something focused in specific areas of health care, e.g. anaesthesia, to an overall approach (see Introduction). However, is this overall approach to patient safety really any different from the TQM approaches described here? Comparisons can be made between these approaches, as shown in Table 4.4 which compares the following:

- TQM, as defined by Hackman and Wageman (1995);
- quality improvement in health, as defined by Berwick et al. (1990/2002);
- the fundamentals of a patient safety approach as described by the NPSA (National Patient Safety Agency 2004);
- the patient safety approach as described by the US National Patient Safety Foundation (National Patient Safety Foundation 1998);
- a seminal book on patient safety in the USA (Kohn et al. 2000).

This comparison shows that all these perspectives focus on the motivation and beliefs of individuals in the organization, which define the culture, as well as the behaviour that results from this. The requirement to obtain and analyse appropriate data is clear in all perspectives, although safety perspectives focus on reporting rather than 'measurement for improvement' which is key for quality. All perspectives do, however, emphasize the role of learning and sharing lessons. However, the role of leadership is not explicit in all cases of either quality or safety, and the assumption that the organization consists of a series of interdependent processes is also not mentioned in all perspectives. The quality perspective focuses on customers, and the safety perspective on patients although the translation between these (are all customers patients?) is not discussed or elucidated. The issue of cost is not mentioned at all in the safety perspectives although it is (as is shown by the review of the work of the quality 'gurus') key in quality improvement.

The lesson for patient safety is surely to get 'back to basics', e.g. mostly focused on data and measurement and identify key principles and tools rather than concentrating on a 'total' package which is almost certain to fail – although some might argue that, by definition, patient safety is back to the basics of good patient care. This view is supported by Shapiro (1996):

If you understand the theory behind the tools and realities of your own situation, you will then have a better chance of understanding the appropriate techniques

Table 4.4 Safety and TQM approaches compared

NPSA Seven Steps to Patient Safety (National Patient Safety Agency 2004)	NPSF beliefs (National Patient Safety Foundation 1998)	To Err is Human recommendations (Kohn et al. 2000)	Common themes of TQM (Hackman and Wageman 1995)	Quality Improvement in Health (Berwick et al. 1990/2002)
1. Build a safety culture	Patient safety is central to quality health care as reflected in the Hippocratic Oath: 'Above All, Do No Harm'. Continued improvement in patient safety is attainable only through establishing a culture of trust, honesty, integrity and open communications.	Patient safety programs should provide strong, clear and visible attention to safety;	Employees naturally care about the quality of the work they do and will take initiatives to improve it	Total employee involvement is crucial
2. Lead and support your staff	Implicit in 'culture' above	Implicit in 'culture' above	Quality is ultimately the responsibility of senior management	Implicit in 'culture' above
3. Integrate your risk management activity	An integrated body of scientific knowledge and the infrastructure to support its development are essential to advance patient safety significantly.		Organizations are systems of interdependent parts	

Continued overleaf

Table 4.4 (*Continued*)

NPSA Seven Steps to Patient Safety (National Patient Safety Agency 2004)	NPSF beliefs (National Patient Safety Foundation 1998)	To Err is Human recommendations (Kohn et al. 2000)	Common themes of TQM (Hackman and Wageman 1995)	Quality Improvement in Health (Berwick et al. 1990/2002)
4. Promote reporting		Patient safety programs should implement non-punitive systems for reporting and analysing errors within their organizations;	Focus on work processes Manage by 'fact' i.e. systematically collected data Use of scientific methods to monitor performance and identify areas for performance improvement	The modern approach to quality is thoroughly grounded in scientific and statistical thinking Productive work is accomplished through processes The main source of quality defects is problems in the process Quality control should focus on the most vital processes
5. Involve and communicate with patients and the public	Patient involvement in continuous learning and constant communication of information between care givers, organizations and the general public will improve patient safety.		Explicit identification and measurement of customer requirements Creation of supplier partnerships	Sound customer-supplier relationships are absolutely necessary for sound quality management

6. Learn and share safety lessons	The system of health care is fallible and requires fundamental change to sustainably improve patient safety.	Patient safety programs should establish interdisciplinary team training programs for providers that incorporate proven methods of team training, such as simulation. Patient safety programs should incorporate well-understood safety principles, such as standardizing and simplifying equipment, supplies, and processes	Analyse variability Learning and continuous improvement Use of cross-functional teams to identify and solve quality problems Use process management approaches to enhance team effectiveness	Understanding the variability of processes is a key to improving quality
7. Implement solutions to prevent harm	Prevention of patient injury, through early and appropriate response to evident and potential problems, is the key to patient safety.	Cost not covered here		
Cost not covered here	Cost not covered here	Quality is less costly to an organization than poor workmanship	Poor quality is costly New organizational structures can help achieve quality improvement Quality management employs three basic, closely interrelated activities: quality planning, quality control and quality improvement

and of knowing how to tailor them to the unique needs and opportunities facing your company.

An excellent review of the UK situation and the potential levers for change in patient safety is provided by Lewis and Fletcher (2005), which highlights the dangers of a top-down rational approach to policy-making and implementation.

The role of people and culture

As quality management approaches were developed in service organizations, the nature of services and the interest in the field from a variety of academic sources led to a tension between 'hard' (systems) approaches and 'soft' (people/culture) issues (Wilkinson 1992). Concerns about the TQM movement stemmed from its promotion as a universal panacea, regardless of context, its disinclination to 'refer to previous management literature – or, indeed, to reference anything outside of the quality management field' (Wilkinson and Willmott 1995), and the 'strong evidence that quality management did not achieve its objectives' (Wilkinson and Brown 2003). At its extreme, perhaps, this developing view describes the quality literature as taking 'an evangelical line that excludes traditions and empirical data that fail to confirm its faith' (Wilkinson and Willmott 1995), a criticism sometimes made of organizations today who promote a single approach.

The gradual emergence of a field comprised largely of research prescribing 'solutions' was also a driving force for this development. Those promoting TQM (or its derivatives) later in the 1990s were able to develop an approach which included more about the impact on employees (Webb 1995) rather than the positivistic perspective of many of the quality 'gurus' who developed means of getting hard information about organizational processes. It is argued that the implementation of TQM depends on people and that a failure of both HR policies and lack of integration of HR and TQM may be to blame. It appears to be taken for granted by the quality 'gurus' that employees will welcome, and be committed to, approaches that minimize unproductive activity and enable them to take a pride in what is produced. However, it is argued that while this is done within the context of a hierarchical relationship between management and employees, the benefits from quality improvement will be limited. The emphasis of quality management on systems rather than individuals may also lead to poor 'buy-in' of the relevant concepts.

Issues that are specifically related to HR and TQM include (Wilkinson and Brown 2003):

- employee involvement (fundamental to TQM);
- training and education (for both tools and the overall approach);
- selection of staff;
- appraisal (with the traditional approach being one of the 'deadly diseases' identified by Deming (1986));
- pay (a controversial area for TQM but seen as fundamental to HR);
- employee well-being (which links to the concept of internal customers in TQM);

- industrial relations (which are affected by the changes required by a TQM approach);
- employment security (which can be perceived as one demonstration of the value put on people by the organization).

Coupled with this increasing emphasis on 'human factors' has come a recognition that organizational culture and change also have a part to play. The culture change aspects, where a 'quality culture' is one 'whereby everyone in the organization shares a commitment to continuous improvement aimed at customer satisfaction' (Wilkinson and Brown, 2003), are seen by both HR and TQM as important, although HR might acknowledge more readily the complexities of culture change, and believe that culture cannot be 'managed' (Schein 1985). The involvement of top management, use of teamwork and the ability to foster innovation were shown to be important in quality improvement (Parker et al. 1999), and a participative, flexible, risk-taking culture was significantly related to the implementation of quality improvement in another study (Shortell et al. 1995).

The learning from this aspect of quality is clear for patient safety – the many exhortations to develop a 'safety culture' need to take into account the complexities of culture and the debates about whether it can be 'managed' (see Chapter 13). However, the 'people' implications are broader than culture, relating to individual employment arrangements, and need to take into account both individuals and systems and recognize the impact of many of the factors described above. TQM as a field is much more advanced in attempting to change the way that organizations and individuals operate, and patient safety would do well to review the lessons already learned the hard way by many organizations.

What does quality contribute to safety?

There are a number of areas where quality management may be able to contribute to patient safety, and the research which supports its development, in line with the needs identified by those at the forefront of this area (Lilford 2002). In order to locate these firmly in the healthcare context, the points made by Berwick (Berwick et al. 1990/2002) in terms of comparing 'what we knew in 1990' (when IHI was established) and 'what we now know that we wished we had known then' are used as a structure (shown in italics below).

It was known in 1990 that quality improvement tools can work in health care, but more recent experience has shown that spending too much time analysing processes can slow the pace of change. Teams can enter the PDCA cycle in several places. Tools are important in their place, but not a very good entry point for improvement. So for patient safety this means that using tools may not necessarily or automatically improve safety as the quality 'gurus' identified in their work focusing on overall approaches. However, given that tools such as root cause analysis (RCA) and FMEA are being relatively easily transferred to health care, it seems likely that there are others which could also provide benefit; design of experiments, policy deployment, quality costing and mistake proofing are some examples. There is also potential in the seven management tools as more qualitative data is used to support the systematic quantitative data that have been the focus of much patient safety research to date.

Cross-functional teams have been acknowledged as valuable in improving healthcare processes, but more recent learning has shown that achieving action is more important than achieving buy-in. The process owner concept from industry is helpful here. In terms of patient safety, therefore, effective teamwork will only result from explicit consideration of the 'people' aspects of improvement – putting people together does not make a workable team. The relative lack of attention to the 'people' factors is cited by some as the main reason for the lack of spread and sustaining of TQM (Parker et al. 1999). The involvement of clinical professionals here is also vital.

Improvement is often said to be a matter of changing the process, not blaming the people, but it is now clear that the shift of blame from individuals to processes is not 100 per cent. There are limits to a blame-free culture, but perhaps not to a process-minded culture. We know in terms of patient safety that culture is important. The exhortations from patient safety proponents to create a 'safety culture' sound as hollow as those proposing a 'quality culture' in the 1980s, unless they consider the complexity of culture (Mannion et al. 2005) and how it may link to changes in performance. The quality movement believes that there are limits to a blame-free culture.

Data useful for quality improvement abound in health care but measurement is very difficult for health care, which seems far behind other industries. Balanced scorecards are helpful and IT is essential. In terms of patient safety, data analysis is vital, as demonstrated in several chapters of this book, and is not unproblematic. Centralized reporting systems utilizing IT are a valuable step in this direction. The use of various tools is also important and dependent on good data, but on its own will not be sufficient for improvement. Data need to reflect the factors 'that contribute to safety shortcomings' (Lewis and Fletcher 2005).

In 1990 Berwick and colleagues believed that quality improvement methods are fun to use – their more recent learning has shown that there need to be consequences for not being involved in improvement (not improving should not be an option). This requires detailed understanding of human motivation and relationships, which can be supported by psychology and human resources research. This is not a simple factor to understand or influence and is as applicable to patient safety as quality management.

Costs of poor quality have long been acknowledged to be high, and savings may be within reach but it is now clear that waste is pervasive in health care, and improvement is the best way to save money. Despite the emphasis put on this by the quality 'gurus', it has not been a major emphasis of quality improvement approaches in the West. Safety seems to be going the same way – there are believed to be higher motives for improving quality and safety, focused on the patient experience, with effects on cost being secondary despite increasing cost focus in both US and UK health systems (see Table 4.4).

Involving doctors in improvement is difficult, and more recently it has become clear that doctors are not well prepared to lead people. Doctors can (and are) learning new skills to supplement their medical training, not to replace it. In terms of patient safety an understanding of the clinical perspective (see Chapter 1) is key and improvements in patient safety require the involvement of everyone in the healthcare system. There must be a recognition that doctors and managers operate within different paradigms, stemming from their basic beliefs about evidence and motivation for action, which will affect their involvement in change of any form (Degeling et al. 2003) and that reluctance to become involved in improvement may not be due to the improvement initiative but to broader issues.

Non-clinical processes drew early attention when quality improvement was first formalized within healthcare but now it is clear that clinical outcomes are critical. This is the 'core business' of health care and focus on clinical factors achieves buy-in from all health professionals. For patient safety, this means that systems of measurement and key processes need to focus on outcomes – something that was also identified as a danger with TQM (Shapiro 1996) – 'has process taken over purpose?'. To some extent this can be achieved by integration of patient safety in routine practice (Lewis and Fletcher 2005), just as making 'quality everyone's business' was a key tenet of quality improvement. Some would not agree that this is applicable in health care (Wilson 2000) and the same attitudes might also extend to patient safety.

Early work on quality improvement showed that healthcare organizations may need a broader definition of quality, and we now know that these must include the whole patient experience – not just clinical outcomes and costs. In terms of patient safety, definitions need to be broad, but spending too many resources on definition at the expense of research and development is not going to actually improve patient safety.

In health care, as in industry, the fate of quality improvement is first of all in the hands of leaders but it is now clearer that the executive leader doesn't always have to be the driver of change. This is especially true at the start of improvement, but achieving system-level improvement does require senior commitment. There will need to be some system-wide and top-down commitment to patient safety, even if improvement does not start there, and there are things that can be learned from quality improvement at this top level (Edwards 2005). It is difficult to imagine how the need to 'create an environment receptive to change' (Lewis and Fletcher 2005) which is seen as essential for patient safety, can be done without effective leadership.

Even the extensive research and empirical evidence about quality improvement does not automatically translate to improved practice – this requires individual and organizational learning, and changes in culture. There is no reason why the same should not apply to patient safety, which is in many ways inextricably linked to quality improvement. Knowledge on its own is not enough: 'the world is now much more knowledgeable about the quality and safety of health care. It is not yet clear that it is any wiser' (Moss 2004).

Note

1   See www.ihi.org

Box 4.1 Key points

- Quality in general, quality in health care, and its relationship to patient safety are not areas about which there is universal agreement on definition, despite a substantial and growing literature in each area.
- There are a wide variety of tools which can be used for quality improvement, which were developed and used by a series of quality 'gurus', some of which are being used to improve patient safety.
- The concept of quality developed from the work of the gurus to be an over-arching 'strategy' for an organization, epitomized by TQM, and which has much in common with approaches being taken to patient safety.
- The importance of people and organizational culture developed in the latter stages of TQM and is similarly viewed as important in patient safety, which could learn much from the 'failure' of quality initiatives because these factors were under-emphasized.
- quality improvement can contribute to patient safety in a variety of areas:

  - the application of improvement tools – although on their own they do not constitute improvement;
  - the role of teamworking and professionals;
  - the role of the process;
  - the effective use of data for improvement, not just measurement, and its relationship to outcomes;
  - the cost of quality and safety;
  - the impact of the organization's leaders, even if a top-down approach is not adopted.

References

Apkon, M., Leonard, J., Probst, L., DeLizio, L. and Vitale, R. (2004) Design of a safer approach to intravenous drug infusions: failure mode effects analysis, *Quality and Safety in Health Care*, 13(4): 265–71.

Bendell, T., Penson, R. and Carr, S. (1995) The quality gurus – their approaches described and considered, *Managing Service Quality*, 5(6): 44–8.

Benneyan, J.C., Lloyd, R.C. and Plsek, P.E. (2003) Statistical process control as a tool for research and healthcare improvement, *Quality and Safety in Health Care*, 12(6): 458–64.

Berry, L.L., Zeithaml, V.A. and Parasuraman, A. (1985) Quality counts in services too, *Business Horizons*, 28(3): 44–52.

Berwick, D. (1989) Continuous improvement as an ideal in healthcare, *New England Journal of Medicine*, 320: 53–6.

Berwick, D., Godfrey, A.B. and Roessner, J. (1990/2002) *Curing Health Care*. San Francisco: Jossey-Bass.

Boaden, R.J., Harvey, G., Proudlove, N., Greatbanks, R., Shephard, A. and Moxham, C. (2005) Quality Improvement: Theory and Practice in the NHS, unpublished report, Manchester.

Camp, R.C. (1989) *Benchmarking: The Search for Industry Best Practice that Leads to Superior Performance*. Milwaukee: ASQC Quality Press.

Carson, P.P., Lanier, P.A., Carson, K.D. and Birkenmeier, B.J. (1999) A historical perspective on fad adoption and abandonment, *Journal of Management History*, 5(6): 320–30.

Clarke, C.L, Reed, J., Wainwright, D., McClelland, S., Swallow, V., Harden, J., Walton, G. and Walsh, A. (2004) The discipline of improvement: something old, something new? *Journal of Nursing Management*, 12: 85–96.

Committee on Quality Health Care in America and Institute of Medicine (2001) *Crossing the Quality Chasm*. Washington, DC: Institute of Medicine.

Cooper, J.B., Sorensen, A.V., Anderson, S.M., Zipperer, L.A., Blum, L.N. and Blim, J.F. (2001) *Current Research on Patient Safety in the United States*. Chicago: National Patient Safety Foundation.

Crosby, P. (1979) *Quality is Free*. New York: McGraw-Hill.

Dale, B.G. (ed.) (2003) *Managing Quality*. Oxford: Blackwell.

Degeling, P., Maxwell, S., Kennedy, J. and Coyle, B. (2003) Medicine, management, and modernisation: a 'danse macabre'? *British Medical Journal*, 326(7390): 649–52.

Deming, W.E. (1986) *Out of the Crisis*. Center of Advanced Engineering Study, Cambridge, MA: MIT Press.

Donabedian, A. (1987) Commentary on some studies of the quality of care, *Health Care Financing Review*, Annual Supplement: 75.

Edwards, N. (2005) Can quality improvement be used to change the wider healthcare system? *Quality and Safety in Health Care*, 14(2): 75.

Feigenbaum, A. (1961) *Total Quality Control*. New York: McGraw-Hill.

Grol, R., Baker, R. and Moss, F. (eds) (2004) *Quality Improvement Research: Understanding the Science of Change in Health Care*. London: BMJ Books.

Groonroos, C. (1984) *Strategic Management and Marketing in the Service Sector*. London: Chartwell-Bratt.

Hackman, J.R. and Wageman, R. (1995) Total quality management: empirical, conceptual and practical issues, *Administrative Science Quarterly*, 40(2): 309–42.

Huczynski, A. (1993) *Management Gurus*. London: Routledge.

Iles, V. and Sutherland, K. (2001) *Organizational Change: A Review for Health Care Managers, Professionals and Researchers*. London: NHS Co-ordinating Centre for NHS Service Delivery and Organisation R&D.

Ishikawa, K. (1979) *Guide to Total Quality Control*. Tokyo: Asian Productivity Organization.

Jick, H. (1974) Drugs – remarkably toxic, *New England Journal of Medicine*, 291: 768–70.

Joint Commission on Accreditation of Healthcare Organizations (2005) Failure mode effect and criticality analysis, http://www.jcaho.org/accredited+organizations/patient+safety/fmeca/index.htm (accessed 11 Mar. 2005).

Juran, J. (ed.) (1951) *The Quality Control Handbook*. New York: McGraw-Hill.

Kaiser Permanente (2005) SBAR Technique for communication: a situational briefing model. http://www.ihi.org/IHI/Topics/PatientSafety/SafetyGeneral/Tools/SBARTechnique for CommunicationASituationalBriefingModel.htm (accessed 11 Mar. 2005).

Kohn, L.T., Corrigan, J.M. and Donaldson, M.S. (eds) (2000) *To Err is Human: Building a Safer Health System*. Washington, DC: National Academy Press.

Kolesar, P.J. (1993) The relevance of research on statistical process control to the total quality movement, *Journal of Engineering and Technology Management*, 10(4): 317–38.

Langley, G.J., Nolan, K.M., Nolan, T.W., Norman, C.L. and Provost, L.P. (1996) *The Improvement Guide*, San Francisco: Jossey-Bass.

Larson, J.S. and Muller, A. (2002/3) Managing the quality of healthcare, *Journal of Health and Health Services Administration*, 25(3/4): 261–80.

Lewis, R.Q. and Fletcher, M. (2005) Implementing a national strategy for patient safety: lessons from the National Health Service in England, *Quality and Safety in Health Care*, 14(2): 135–9.

Lilford, R.J. (2002) Patient safety research: does it have legs? *Quality and Safety in Health Care*, 11: 113–14.

Mannion, R., Davies, H.T.O. and Marshall, M.N. (2005) *Cultures for Performance in Health Care*. Maidenhead: Open University Press.

Maxwell, R.J. (1984) Quality assessment in health, *British Medical Journal*, 288: 1470–2.

McBryde, V.E. (1986) In today's market: quality is best focal point for upper management, *Industrial Engineering*, 18(7): 51–5.

McLaughlin, C.P. and Simpson, K.N. (1999) Does TQM/CQI work in healthcare? in C.P. McLaughlin and A.D. Kaluzny (eds) *Continuous Quality Improvement in Health Care: Theory, Implementation and Applications*. Gaithersburg: Aspen.

McNulty, T. and Ferlie, E. (2002) *Reengineering Health Care: The Complexities of Organizational Transformation*. Oxford: Oxford University Press.

Merry, M.D. and Crago, M.G. (2001) The past, present and future of health care quality, *Physician Executive*, 27(5): 30–6.

Moss, F. (2004) Quality and safety in health care: plus ça change, plus ça ne reste plus la même chose, *Quality and Safety in Health Care*, 13: 5–6.

Moss, F. and Barach, P. (2002) Quality and safety in health care: a time of transition, *Quality and Safety in Health Care*, 11(1): 1.

National Patient Safety Agency (2004) *Seven Steps to Patient Safety*. London: NPSA.

National Patient Safety Foundation (1998) About the Foundation http://www.npsf.org/html/about_npsf.html (accessed 11 Mar. 2005).

Nielsen, D.M., Merry, M.D., Schyve, P.M. and Bisognano, M. (2004) Can the gurus' concepts cure healthcare? *Quality Progress*, 37(9): 25–6.

Parker, V.A., Wubbenhorst, W., Young, G., Desai, K. and Charns, M. (1999) Implementing quality improvement in hospitals: the role of leadership and culture, *American Journal of Medical Quality*, 14(1): 64–9.

Plsek, P. (1999) Quality improvement methods in clinical medicine, *Pediatrics*, 103(1): 203–14.

Reason, J. (1997) *Managing the Risk of Organizational Accidents*. Ashgate: Aldershot.

Reason, J. and Wreathall, J. (2005) Checklist for assessing institutional resilience. http://www.ihi.org/IHI/Topics/PatientSafety/SafetyGeneral/Tools/ChecklistForAssessingInstitutionalResilience.htm (accessed 11 Mar. 2005).

Reeves, C.A. and Bednar, D.A. (1994) Defining quality: alternatives and implications, *The Academy of Management Review*, 19(3): 419–56.

Resar, R.K., Rozich, J.D. and Classen, D. (2003) Methodology and rationale for the measurement of harm with trigger tools, *Quality and Safety in Health Care*, 12(6): 39ii–45.

Schein, E.H. (1985) *Organizational Culture and Leadership*. Oxford: Jossey-Bass.

Seddon, J. (2003) *Freedom from Command and Control*. Buckingham: Vanguard Press.

Senders, J.W. (2004) FMEA and RCA: the mantras of modern risk management, *Quality and Safety in Health Care*, 13(4): 249–50.

Sexton, B., Thomas, E., Helmreich, R. and Pronovost, P. (2005) The Safety Climate Survey. http://www.ihi.org/IHI/Topics/PatientSafety/MedicationSystems/Tools/Safety+Climae-+Survey+%28IHI+Tool%29.htm (accessed 11 Mar. 2005).

Shapiro, E. (1996) *Fad Surfing in the Boardroom*. Oxford: Capstone Publishing.

Shewhart, W.A. (1931) *Economic Control of Quality of Manufactured Product*. New York: Van Nostrand.

Shingo, S. (1986) *Zero Quality Control: Source Inspection and the Poka-Yoke System*. Cambridge MA: Productivity Press.

Shortell, S.M., O'Brien, J.L., Carman, J.M., Foster, R.W., Hughes, E.F.X, Boerstler, H. and O'Connor, E.J. (1995) Assessing the impact of continuous quality improvement/total quality management: concept versus implementation, *Health Services Research*, 30(2): 377–401.

Taguchi, G. (1986) *Introduction to Quality Engineering*. New York: Asian Productivity Organization.

Vincent, C. (1997) Risk, safety, and the dark side of quality, *British Medical Journal*, 314(7097): 1775–6.

Vinzant, J.C. and Vinzant, D.H. (1999) Strategic management spin-offs of the Deming approach, *Journal of Management History*, 5(8): 516–31.

Webb, J. (1995) Quality management and the management of quality in A. Wilkinson and H. Willmott (eds) *Making Quality Critical*. London: Routledge.

Wilkinson, A. (1992) The other side of quality: soft issues and the human resource dimension, *Total Quality Management*, 3(3): 323–9.

Wilkinson, A. and Willmott, H. (eds) (1995) *Making Quality Critical*. London: Routledge.

Wilkinson, A.J. and Brown, A. (2003) Managing human resources for quality management, in B.G. Dale (ed.) *Managing Quality*. Oxford: Blackwell, pp. 177–202.

Wilson, L. (2000) 'Quality is everyone's business': why this approach will not work in hospitals, *Journal of Quality in Clinical Practice*, 20(4): 131–5.

Wright, A. (1997) Public service quality: lessons not learned, *Total Quality Management*, 8(5): 313–21.

5

Technology, informatics and patient safety

Paul Beatty

A few years ago I went to a multidisciplinary conference on approaches to patient safety. One of the invited speakers was an experienced engineer, from a university engineering department with a deserved reputation in medical engineering. With a bright smile on his face and considerable enthusiasm he announced to the company that engineering could solve all their safety problems, all they needed to do was ask. As the people around me sniggered or smiled indulgently, I inwardly groaned at his naïvety, whilst at the same time sympathizing with his dilemma. For while it is clear that the biggest advances in patient safety are most likely to come about through the insights of the human factor sciences – sociology, psychology, management and information science – it would be a brave person who would say that technology does not have a bearing on promoting patient safety.

What has been the engineering perspective of patient safety?

In most areas of engineering, including medical engineering, the traditional approach has been to provide more and more 'defence in depth', by which I mean the duplication or replacement of human activities by technology. While there are many examples of 'defence in depth', quintessentially it has been provided by utilizing automatic control systems and where possible by replacing 'unreliable' human operators. Where automatic control has not been possible, it has resulted in technology being used to supply more and more sources of information that can be used for control by a human operator. This treats the 'human in the loop' as if they were the equivalent of an automatic control system.

This approach developed imperceptibly throughout the late nineteenth and early twentieth centuries, particularly in railways and latterly in aviation. So there is a conceptual link between such things as audible alarms on patient monitoring equipment in the ITU and signalling on Brunel's Great Western Railway, although the technologies used are radically different. However, since the Second World War two things have greatly accelerated the process:

- the introduction of industries, such as nuclear power generation, where the technology itself was inherently dangerous and could not be implemented except using remote control technologies;

- the growing dominance of electronic control methods, culminating in the use of computer control which is able to integrate large numbers of potential information streams or inputs.

Extending this traditional role for technology continues. For instance, it can be argued that one of the motivations behind the development of computer-based medical decision support systems for diagnosis is concern about the fallibility of clinical judgement. No doubt in the increasingly litigious and compensation-oriented culture of the USA, the UK and elsewhere, such pressure will continue to exist. Thus, many medical engineers will continue to be attracted by the dream of 'engineering out' human error by using ever more powerful computers, with ever more subtle reasoning engines, to eliminate or restrict the area of discretion of the human in the loop. However, even in engineering terms alone, there are multiple limitations to this approach.

First, it ignores the fact that there are very few situations in medicine where a machine capable of being controlled by a computer can be used to dispense the treatment to the patient. Administration of treatment requires a human being, susceptible to human error.

Second, even in the limited situations where automatic control might be possible, attempts to implement it are often foiled by the biological variability between patients. For instance, in the case of control of neuromuscular blockading drugs used during anaesthesia to relax the skeletal muscles of patients to aid surgery, it is possible to implement closed loop control of the administration of the drugs using an infusion pump (Ting et al. 2004). This is possible because there is a clear independent signal of the effect of the drugs derived from the response of muscles to electrical stimulation of the nerves supplying them. It is also possible to produce very sophisticated computer models to control the administration. However, even small degrees of difference in patient response can easily make the quality of administration of blockade in an individual patient inferior to that given by a clinician.

Third, there is also the overhead in time on busy operating lists of setting up the equipment required, for little or no gain in terms of quality of care, in all but exceptional cases where human control is difficult. The technique, if it is used at all, is only used for the rare exceptional case.

Fourth, since system safety is highly dependent on the design of the system, software reliability and other issues of implementation, errors by the designer and or the design of the system itself become critical.

The human factors disadvantages of the 'defence in depth' approach are similarly daunting. Since the role of the operator can easily become to control those functions that the designer of the system cannot think of a way of automating, 'defence in depth' systems may only call the operator into action at critical moments. Hours of boredom followed by seconds of panic are likely to lead to poor vigilance even in the most dedicated operator. Further, 'defence in depth' systems tend to be complex and thus opaque, making appropriate human intervention difficult and adversely affecting efficiency of training. Automatic control functions can also closely couple in time separate events leading to a cascade that the operators have no time to respond to.

What does an engineering perspective contribute to patient safety?

Traditional engineering attitudes and modes of approaching problems in patient safety may not be particularly helpful or sit easily with the insights of the human factor sciences. Nevertheless, engineering brings techniques and methodological attitudes that can be of great help not only in considering technology's role in promoting patient safety but in promoting patient safety in general.

Project planning and task analysis

Engineering, in particular civil engineering, has always had to deal with large-scale projects where many complex and disparate processes have to be interlocked, and where people and material have to be co-ordinated. Engineering has thus been in the forefront of the use and development of project planning techniques, e.g. PERT, Critical Path Analysis, etc. (Burke 2003). The application of these techniques is now standard engineering operating procedure, even in small projects involving lesser quantities of material than major civil engineering projects. Project planning is used both to define and manage the progress of the project by dealing with the sequence of tasks that have to be performed to get the project done, identifying the tasks that may hold up overall progress of the project (those on the critical path), allocating resources to achieve the project objectives in a given time and setting concrete achievements (milestones) that indicate how the project is progressing.

Many of the concepts in project planning owe much to ergonomics in general and behavioural approaches in particular. This reflects a time and motion study approach. Thus, the inspiration for these techniques has come not simply from engineering, and aspects of techniques used sit on the border between engineering and the human factor sciences, as do other less project-oriented techniques. Task Analysis and, to a lesser extent, Root Cause Analysis are techniques in this position.

Task Analysis shares with Project Planning the analysis of a complex sequence of events task by task. They both ask the same basic questions: 'What is being done?' and 'How are these tasks accomplished?' Task Analysis is finding direct application in some engineering problems such as the design and control of human–computer interfaces (Curran et al. 2004). However, the tasks in Task Analysis are much more cognitive in nature and lead to an understanding of what is happening through a cognitive model or another type of description. Project Planning, on the other hand, assumes that we know or can describe what is to be done in a way commonly understood by those who will perform those tasks.

Engineering brings to the process of Task Analysis the lesson that any execution of a plan based upon it requires that everyone who is to execute that plan must look at the problem in the same way. Understanding of the plan has to be available at an everyday operational level, as well as at a very high level of overall objectives and at the level of fine detail afforded by Task Analysis.

Planned preventative maintenance

Another insight that engineering can bring to patient safety in general is to emphasize the need for systems that promote patient safety to be maintained and audited regularly in a codified and rigorous way.

Good engineering extends into the area of maintaining the systems it creates, safe and functioning, even after the project is finished. Brunel's first great bridge spans the gorge of the River Avon at Clifton, near Bristol. It is over 200m long and stands 75m above the river. When it was built, it was the longest and highest single span suspension bridge in the world. Thus, its maintenance posed unique difficulties. Brunel's care as an engineer extended to addressing those difficulties and included specifications for tools to enable the maintenance. Some of those tools are still in use today.

In the maintenance of medical equipment in hospitals, best practice has become the use of planned preventative maintenance (MDA 1998). In this process the pieces of equipment to be maintained are placed on an inventory, which includes the routine maintenance cycles recommended by their manufacturers. A schedule of these cycles is included, with instructions on how to do the maintenance and lists of parts required, etc. The philosophy behind the process is described by its name. The equipment is being maintained before it fails and thus the process reduces unexpected failures and increases safety. The process is often controlled using a quality control system such as ISO 9000 (Kent 1993), which includes procedures that record failures of equipment and ensure that the full maintenance history of a piece of equipment can be traced at any time.

In fact, a planned preventative maintenance system is not simply maintaining the equipment; it is as much about maintaining the priority of maintenance in the minds of those who use and maintain the equipment. When combined with a quality control system, it also gives a transparent view of how to operate the system to anyone interested or in need of remembering how to do it.

The lesson for patient safety systems is that, once implemented, how to operate the system and the reasons for operating the system need to be kept fresh in people's minds. The system also needs to be transparent and accessible, both publicly to the group operating the system and privately to individuals who need to refer to it. A standardized procedure for dealing with the system, while it may sound inflexible, supports a consistent approach and helps traceability.

Codification

Historically, engineering has seen safety in many areas as a matter of standardization and codification. In the 1800s in Manchester the weaving industry was powered using high-pressure steam engines. However, there was no standardized method of designing pressure boilers and fatal accidents were common due to explosions. Analysis of the reasons for explosions showed that in many cases it was the weakness of rivets and bolts used in boiler construction that was the root cause of failure. Consequently, in 1841, Joseph Whitworth invented the first standardized range of nuts and bolts, the main feature of which was that screw pitch, thread density and shaft diameter maximized the assembled strength of any joint made with them. The Whitworth thread became adopted as British Standard thread type (BSW) and a de facto world standard through its use in the British Empire. He also ensured accurate construction of Whitworth nuts and bolts, by producing standardized, certificated taps and dies for sale world-wide.

National bodies such as the British Standards Institute (BSI) or international bodies such as the International Standards Organization (ISO), now control the standardization of safety specifications and their promulgation. Standards already include codes controlling how medical instruments are constructed (e.g. the ISO 60601 family of standards on medical device design) which include standards for the design of safety devices such as audible alarms. The argument for their use is similar to the argument for quality standards in planned preventative maintenance, that of ensuring minimum standards and making those standards transparent to users. Since they are arrived at by consensus, they codify what is general to a problem, which may be somewhat limited in the area of patient safety where individualized solutions will probably dominate. However, where a standardized approach can be used, the experience of engineering is that it has distinct benefits, though there are downsides as well.

The GEMS framework: enhancing safety behaviours with technology

In 1987 Reason described the General Error Modelling System (GEMS) to provide a conceptual framework within to locate the origins of basic human error types (Reason 1987). It is summarized in Figure 5.1. GEMS built on the work of Rasmussen (1986) and Rouse (1981) in dividing responses to a new situation requiring an action, into three levels: skill-based, rule-based and knowledge-based (see Chapter 3). It incorporated the concepts that it is the nature of the human mind that it cannot deal with more than a few pieces of knowledge at any one time, regardless of how many are required to make an accurate decision and that we try to minimize our cognitive workload or strain when making decisions. Thus, we are predisposed to look for pre-packaged solutions to problems rather than go through the cognitive effort of devising an original solution from first principles.

Consider the GEMS-based explanation of the reaction of an anaesthetist to a blood oxygen (SpO$_2$) alarm during anaesthesia. By their actions any operator then tries to return the system to a stable state. This is the desired goal state; in our example, no alarm with satisfactory SpO$_2$. The operator will first apply a simple action at the skill-based level, without any real thought. So in our example, they might see the SpO$_2$ connector had come loose and will tighten it. If simple actions taken do not resolve the error state, the operator goes to the rule-based level, in which they consider the general state of the situation, for example, they look at all the patient monitor readings. If the pattern is familiar, they apply a series of actions that have been shown in the past to resolve the situation. This series of actions constitutes the rule to be applied. For instance, they might notice that the inspired oxygen level has dropped and that the inspiratory pressure is zero. This is the pattern of a breathing system disconnection, so the rule to apply is check the breathing system function. Rule-based behaviours are fast and if correctly selected, very effective at resolving

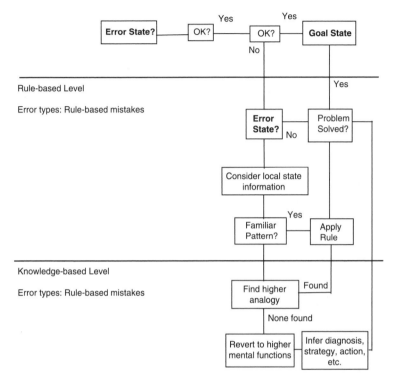

Figure 5.1 The Generic Error Modelling System, GEMS
Source: Reason (1987)

error states. The final stage is knowledge-based behaviour, which requires higher cognitive effort. The operator then has to work out from 'first principles' what is wrong. GEMS suggests that most human factors errors arise because of the selection of the wrong rule by the operator or the failure to realize the rule being applied is inappropriate or to realize that they do not have the required knowledge to synthesize a correct solution.

In the general consideration of the patient safety GEMS has not received much attention. However, in terms of engineering technology to enhance patient safety, it is particularly useful because it suggests that it should be possible to design devices that help nudge people out of the rule-based trap. The question arises if it is a good model in practice. Apart from the theoretical arguments it embodies, there is good phenomenological evidence that it is.

For example, Table 5.1 shows the nature of errors committed by trainee anaesthetists undergoing safety training in an anaesthetic simulator (DeAnda and Gaba

Table 5.1 Nature of unforced errors and their causes analysed using GEMS during anaesthesia simulation

Type of error	per cent	Reason for inducing Rule-based Error
Failure to check	43.9	
Inexperience	41.0	
Inattention	32.7	Denying the operator vital information required to
Fixation	20.5	trigger a move to the knowledge base
Haste	25.8	
Distraction	14.0	
Fatigue	10.8	Not recognizing the need to move to the knowledge base
Not following procedure	6.1	Not using the generic rules

1990). Table 5.1 refers only to errors the trainees spontaneously created, i.e. the critical incidents that developed were not imposed on them as part of the training. Since these critical incidents were generated in a simulator, they could be analysed in depth and the type of error committed identified. More than one error can arise for a single incident so that the total percentages in Table 5.1 can legitimately add up to more than 100 per cent. The third column in Table 5.1 shows that all these types of error, except the last, can be ascribed to the rule-based knowledge-based interface within the GEMS model. The only one that cannot is not following procedures, which is most likely to be a failure of training, basic knowledge or some form of violation, which are deliberate acts performed in contravention of established best practice guidelines (Beatty and Beatty 2004a). While anaesthesia may seem to be an area a long way from patient safety issues such as medication errors, it shows all the characteristics of the human factors error common to critical incident development and has been studied in depth for much longer than most areas in medicine, with detailed critical incident and other studies starting in the 1970s (Cooper et al. 1978).

Table 5.2 shows a summary of behaviours that lead to the self-detection and correction of errors exhibited by operators of complex systems. All these error detection methods fit into the GEMS description and, to a lesser or greater extent, address the rule-based trap problem.

Self-monitoring occurs where the operator performs a more or less systematic check of how the system is performing without an easily defined link to the goal state of the system considered by GEMS. Incremental experiments, on the other hand, are much more deliberative. In most patient safety environments, such actions are likely to be by way of 'thought experiments' since safely adjusting the system to see what might happen is not possible. The standard check is probably the most interesting behaviour under self-monitoring. It consists of a systematic sweep of the available sources of information. The standard check is done at times of crisis but also at times when little is happening, in which case it is a strategy that improves vigilance.

The second type of error detection method is the environmental cue. In anaesthesia and critical care, artificial ventilators emit rhythmic, low volume sounds as they

Table 5.2 Naturally occurring error correction strategies

Error detection method	Example
Self-monitoring	
Automatic actions	Things don't feel right
Incremental experiments	Asking what if or is there a fault
Standard check	Sweep of controls/inputs in a systematic way
Environmental cues	
Audible cues	Background sounds
Forcing functions	Not being able to do things
Other people	
Independent observer	Have you seen that?
Experienced supervisor	Are you aware of that?

push gas in and out of the patient. These sounds readily become background sounds, which are ignored. However, if they change, the anaesthetist immediately becomes aware of the change and is highly likely to check the equipment or initiate a standard check. The other type of environmental cue used is the forcing function. This is a device that physically prevents a dangerous action. If forcing functions are clearly and simply linked to a recognized danger, then they work well. The ideal forcing function in the GEMS context would be a device that stopped a simple false action but also triggered a wider review of the situation.

Finally, we have other people, more exactly, the appearance on the scene of an independent observer who sees what is happening as it is and who is not locked into an inappropriate rule-based view. This person may be a casual arrival on the scene or it may be a person in a formal supervisory role.

The most encouraging thing from an engineering point of view is that it is conceivable that these self-correcting mechanisms can be triggered or enhanced using technology. Such devices might appropriately be termed cognitively ergonomic, or to use the term coined by Rasmussen and Vicente (1987) ecological, fitting into how the operator thinks, not cutting across it.

The challenge of emerging technologies, especially health informatics

The concrete examples I have taken in this chapter have been from anaesthesia and critical care. These are areas where there has been a history of patient safety work and thus it affords useful examples. It is also an area where there is a great deal of computer power in close proximity to the clinician, which allows for the design of technological approaches to patient safety. This is not the case in many areas of medicine where patient safety is important. This situation is about to change with the development of health informatics systems.

Health informatics is an extremely wide and sometimes ill-defined discipline. One working definition is supplied by Protti (2002), 'the study of the nature and principles of information and its application within all aspects of healthcare delivery and promotion'. Areas of application include information systems, medical documentation, signal processing, image processing, medical decision support, telemedicine and molecular bioinformatics. It is predicted that the impact of health informatics will be extensive. For instance in the UK, the National Programme for Information Technology (NPfIT) has the target of connecting over 30,000 GPs in England to almost 300 hospitals and giving patients access to their personal healthcare information, in the next ten years.

While the overall effects of health informatics on health care are not certain, it is clear that the large-scale deployment of computer technology of the programs of the NPfIT, will change the landscape of the medical technology, providing support for new technological approaches to patient safety.

The most obvious effect will be the appearance of personal computing technology in all-medical environments. Since it has become commonplace, the power of the current generation of personal computers is significantly underrated. The average desktop PC with a 3.5 GHz processor, 1 GB of RAM and a 40 GB hard disk is capable of performing very sophisticated calculations on its own, which might be the basis of many possible technological approaches to enhancing patient safety. However, that PC will not be alone. Its primary informatics function will be a gateway to wider networks to provide the user with connectivity to distant sites or to wide-area networks within a single site such as a hospital. This offers anyone designing technology to enhance patient safety access to a lot of comparative information and also to a lot of complementary computer power through grid technologies. These are a type of parallel and distributed computer system that enables the sharing, selection, and aggregation of geographically distributed individual computers into a single computing resource, so that the single problems may be solved dynamically at runtime, depending on the individual computer's availability, capability, performance, cost, and grid users' quality-of-service requirements.

There will also be the development and integration into such systems of Personal Digital Assistant (PDA) technologies, which will be used by individual clinicians within hospitals, while engaged in normal clinical duties, to perform tasks such as ordering prescriptions, checking laboratory test results, or viewing patient-oriented data such as operating theatre lists.

Thus, the technological environment that health informatics will bring, will facilitate technological initiatives to enhance patient safety that are computer-based, information-driven, possibly mathematically intensive and can be delivered in a very personalized manner.

What do new engineering approaches bring to patient safety implementation?

The concept of technologies that trigger natural methods of error correction has been discussed in the previous section. There will also be a need to develop new algorithms and approaches to errors accessible through the health informatics infrastructure. However, the most interesting line of enquiry concerns the possible use of persuasive technologies.

Persuasive technologies

Noting that people often treat computers in ways that suggest that they sometimes see them as surrogate humans (shouting at them, talking to them, etc.), Fogg (1999) has suggested that computer systems may be designed to be persuasive, i.e. designed to change people's attitudes and behaviours. He has gone on to propose that to do this they should perform one or more of three roles in a Functional Triad of Captology (Computers as Persuasive Technologies), summarized in Figure 5.2. This triad suggests that to be persuasive, technologies should interact with users in one of three ways, as:

- Tools: which assist the person in behaving in the desired way
- Medium: which allows experience of behaviours
- Social Actors: where technologies form relationships with users.

In the context of the triad, many of the examples given above, coming out of the GEMS analysis, are Tools. In a device as Medium, the main intention would be to allow the user to experience the behaviour, investigate underlying cause and effect relationships or help people rehearse correct behaviours. For instance, a computer program, running on the operating theatre computer that would allow the anaesthetist to explore potential new settings for the ventilator might be a medium-based approach to the problem of ventilation optimization addressed in a more limited way using incremental experiments. Such a 'what if' device would require an element of simulation. In fact, the use of simulation as Medium can be extended greatly, either in the form of the sort of realistic simulation of operating theatre environments given by mannikin-based anaesthesia simulators or in simulations of clinical situations that rehearse how a team of staff work together.

Devices as Social Actors is easily the most difficult leg of the triad to envisage and the most fascinating. If persuasive technologies that work can be designed in this area, it is here that they will have the most impact on patient safety. However, do people

Tools

Increasing capability
- Making the target behaviour easier
- Leading people through a process
- Perform motivating calculations

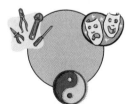

Social Actors

Creating relationships
- Rewarding people with positive feedback
- Modelling a target behaviour
- Providing social support

Medium

Provides experience of behaviour outcome
- Allows exploration of cause and effect relationships
- Providing experience of how behaviours emerge
- Helping people rehearse behaviour

Figure 5.2 Fogg's Functional Triad of Captology

form enough of an emotional/relational bond with a computer or similar devices to make persuasive technological social actors possible? Nass and Moon (2000) suggest that this is the case. They find that people respond to computers in a very human way. They respond to politeness and flattery in the way the computer behaves towards them. They differentiate in their own behaviour if the computer has female or male gender. They also think of computers as 'team mates', performing better with computers they have used before. A bond of this type means that given the right method of presentation, the computer could apply social influences to the user. A case study of a persuasive approach to problems of safety compliance suggested by a recent study is presented in Box 5.1.

Box 5.1 A case study: the anaesthetist's friend

In a recent study (Beatty and Beatty 2004a) we found that anaesthetists reported that, in violation of recognized safety guidelines they were likely not to perform a safety check of the anaesthetic equipment to be used in their next list, the so-called 'cock-pit' check, under certain circumstances, e.g. if the operating department assistant (ODA) reported that they had already done the check or if they were in a rush. A technological approach to reducing this type of violation might be to make anaesthetic machines capable of doing their own self-checks automatically. However, that might generate an assumption by anaesthetists that because it *could be done* it *had been* done.

The essence of the guideline is to make sure the anaesthetists themselves take responsibility for the check and look analytically at its results. Thus, there needs to be an individual component to the check. We have suggested (Beatty and Beatty 2004b) that each anaesthetist should be given a PDA capable of being plugged into the anaes-thetic machine. The PDA would be capable of triggering an automatic 'cock-pit' check. This check could be triggered by an ODA if required. However, in performing the check the PDA would gather the data from this check, report the findings and insist that the anaesthetist sign off the check on the PDA to prove that it had been done before proceeding with the anaesthetic. That sign-off would become part of the records of all patients on the list.

Once the interfaces have been established, other functions addressing other potential error safety issues can be added to the system. These are summarized below, divided up using the triad:

Tools
• for pre-operative data taking by nurses speeding pre-operative visits;
• to provide advanced alarm functions during anaesthesia;
• to provide automatic pre-equipment checking.

Medium
• allows review and rehearsal of possible critical incidents and violations;
• provides up-to-date best practice advice.

Social Actor
• provides private feedback on overall critical incident and violation performance.

Box 5.2 Key points

- The traditional role of technology in patient safety has been to provide 'defence in depth' where automatic control systems are used when possible and humans replaced by more 'reliable' technology.
- However, 'engineering out' human error is problematic, even in engineering terms, and there are additional human factors disadvantages to this approach.
- The engineering approaches of project planning and task analysis, planned preventative maintenance and codification can contribute to patient safety.
- The General Error Modelling System (GEMS) provides a helpful framework for understanding how safety behaviours can be enhanced by technology.
- To support patient safety in the future, ecological approaches to technologies will be essential and persuasive technologies will be desirable, as they may enable behaviour change.
- Engineering on its own can never provide a total 'solution' to patient safety issues but in partnership with human factors scientists there is immense potential.

References

Beatty, P. and Beatty, S. (2004a) Anaesthetists' intentions to violate safety guidelines, *Anaesthesia*, 59: 528–40.

Beatty, P. and Beatty, S. (2004b) Designing an anaesthetist's friend: Can persuasive technology improve patient safety? In J. Jan, J. Kozumplik and I. Provaznik (eds) *Biosignal 2004*. Brno, Czech Republic: Vutium Press, pp. 431–3.

Burke, R. (2003) *Project Management: Planning and Control Techniques*. 4th edn. Chichester: John Wiley and Sons.

Cooper, J., Newbower, R., Long, C. and McPeek, P. (1978) Preventable anaesthesia mishaps: a study of human factors, *Anaesthesiology*, 49: 399–406.

Curran, E., Sykacek, P., Stokes, M., Roberts, S.J., Penny, W., Johnsrude, I. and Owen, A.M. (2004) Cognitive tasks for driving a brain-computer interfacing system: a pilot study, *IEEE Transactions on Neural Systems and Rehabilitation Engineering*, 12: 48–54.

DeAnda, A. and Gaba, D. M. (1990) Unplanned incidents during comprehensive anaesthesia simulation, *Anaesthesia and Analgesia*, 71: 77–82.

Fogg, B.J. (1999) Persuasive technologies – now is your chance to decide what they will persuade us to do – and how they'll do it, *Communications of the ACM*, 42: 26–9.

Kent, O. (1993) ISO9000: a quality opportunity, *Byte*, 18: 36.

Nass, C. and Moon, Y. (2000) Machines and mindlessness: social responses to computers, *Journal of Social Issues*, 56: 81–103.

Protti, D. (2002) A proposal to use a balanced scorecard to evaluate Information for Health: an information strategy for the modern NHS (1998–2005), *Computers in Biology and Medicine*, 32: 221–36.

Rasmussen, J. (1986) *Information Processing and Human–Machine Interaction: An Approach to Cognitive Engineering*. New York: Elsevier Science.

Rasmussen, J. and Vicente, K.J. (1987) Cognitive Control of Human Activities: The Implications for Ecological Interface Design. Roskilde, Denmark: RISO Labs.

Reason, J. (1987) Generic error-modeling system (GEMS): a cognitive framework for locating common human error forms. In J. Rasmussen, K. Duncan and J. Leplat (eds) *New Technology and Human Error*. Chichester: John Wiley and Sons, Ltd, pp. 63–83.

Rouse, W.B. (1981) Models of human problem solving: Detection, diagnosis and compensation for system failures. In *Proceedings of the IFAC Conference on Analysis, Design and Evaluation of Man-Machine Systems*. Baden-Baden, FRG: Elsevier.

Ting, C.H., Arnott, R.H., Linkens, D.A. and Angel, A. (2004) Migrating from target-controlled infusion to closed-loop control in general anaesthesia, *Computer Methods and Programs in Biomedicine*, 75: 127–39.

6

Patient safety and the law

Michael A. Jones

For many years, before the concept of risk management began to penetrate practice in the NHS, the law of negligence arguably offered the greatest incentive to patient safety.[1] The simple, probably simplistic, equation was: exercise reasonable care for the safety of patients or find yourself on the receiving end of a writ. In practice, of course, the actual number of claims for negligence is a small percentage of the number of adverse events occurring in the NHS, and the chances of any individual doctor being sued were quite low. Nonetheless, the *threat* of litigation provided the context against which discussions about patient safety took place. The strength of the legal perspective is that the law can subject a single incident of harm to a patient to a detailed scrutiny, and the forensic process can identify, in retrospect, what went wrong in a specific case. But the law's weakness is that it can rarely offer a systematic analysis of the wider causes of harm or how to go about preventing them. The injunction to a potential defendant to 'exercise reasonable care' involves a high level of abstraction which depends on its specific factual context for any real meaning. As a guide to what constitutes safe practice it is almost useless.

This chapter will provide a very brief summary of the major elements of the legal test for negligence; a discussion of the relationship between the law, litigation in general, and medical practice; and, finally, a brief assessment of what the law contributes to patient safety.

The legal perspective – the test for negligence

The test for medical (or 'clinical') negligence was set out in the case of *Bolam* v. *Friern Hospital Management Committee*. Although merely a judge's direction to a jury, and therefore simply an attempt to give non-lawyers a feel for the meaning of negligence in the context of professional liability, the *Bolam* test has been approved by the House of Lords on several occasions, and therefore has significant authoritative status. McNair J explained that the normal test for negligence, is whether the defendant has failed to act reasonably, by reference to the standards of the hypothetical ordinary, reasonable man, or the 'man on the Clapham omnibus':

But where you get a situation which involves the use of some special skill or competence, then the test whether there has been negligence or not is not the test of the man on the Clapham omnibus, because he has not got this special skill. The test is the standard of the ordinary skilled man exercising and professing to have that special skill. A man need not possess the highest expert skill at the risk of being found negligent . . . it is sufficient if he exercises the ordinary skill of an ordinary competent man exercising that particular art.[2]

Thus, there is a margin of error: the lawyer does not guarantee to win the case and the surgeon does not guarantee to 'cure' the patient. Note that this type of statement tends to be made of a particular type of professional practice. Although it may be reasonable for the litigation lawyer or the surgeon to say 'I win some, I lose some', one does not hear an engineer say 'I build bridges, some stay up, some fall down.'

Negligence means a failure to act in accordance with the standards of a reasonably competent professional at the time, provided that it is remembered that there may be one or more perfectly proper standards:

A doctor is not guilty of negligence if he has acted in accordance with a practice accepted as proper by a responsible body of medical men skilled in that particular art . . . Putting it the other way round, a doctor is not negligent, if he is acting in accordance with such a practice, merely because there is a body of opinion that takes a contrary view.[3]

There are a number of issues that need to be teased out of the *Bolam* test. When jury trials were the norm in civil litigation, the issue of whether the defendant had been negligent was for the jury to decide, and so it was treated as a question of fact rather than a question of law. However, jury trials for most civil litigation involving personal injury claims were effectively abolished in the 1960s. There are two stages in the process. First, there must be an assessment by the court of how, in the circumstances, the defendant *ought* to have behaved – what standard of care should he have exercised? This enquiry necessarily involves a normative judgment, which may be conditioned, but should not necessarily be determined, by the expert evidence. The second stage requires a decision about whether on the facts of the case (as determined from the evidence) the defendant's conduct fell below the appropriate standard. This is truly a question of fact, as opposed to a question of law.

In reaching the normative judgment about what standard of care ought to be applied, the courts apply a number of general principles. First, the standard of care expected of the reasonable professional is objective. It does not take account of the subjective attributes of the particular defendant.[4] One consequence of this is that the defendant's inexperience is not a defence – his 'incompetent best' is not good enough.[5] Nor is the standard of care necessarily determined by the average conduct of people in general if that conduct is routinely careless. Similarly, there is no concept of an 'average' standard of care by which a defendant might argue that he has provided an adequate service on average and should not be held liable for the occasions when his performance fell below the norm. No matter how skilled the defendant's conduct was, he will be responsible for even a single occasion when he fell below the standard of reasonable care if damage results from that.[6]

Despite the objective nature of the standard of care, the tort[7] of negligence is fault-based. So if there was no way of anticipating the injury to the claimant, there is no negligence. A defendant will be liable only for foreseeable harm; risks that could not have been foreseen *at the time of the allegedly negligent conduct* are not taken into account.[8] On the other hand, not all foreseeable risks give rise to liability; the defendant's obligation is to exercise *reasonable* care, not take absolute care, and what is reasonable varies with the circumstances. In some circumstances it may be reasonable to ignore a small foreseeable risk. The courts look at the magnitude of the risk of harm, which is a product of two factors: (1) the likely incidence of harm; and (2) the probable severity of any harm that may occur. So if the risk of injury occurring is very small, it may be reasonable simply to ignore the risk, and take no precautions against it;[9] but, on the other hand, if the damage, should it materialize, is likely to be severe, it may be negligent to ignore even a small risk.[10] Also factored into the equation is the defendant's purpose, or reason, for acting in a particular way – a laudable purpose, such as saving life or limb, will justify the taking of greater risk than, say, a simple commercial objective.[11] This is clearly a factor in dealing with medical accidents since the assumption is that medicine is concerned with saving life and limb. There are limits to this, however. For example, there is no point in a fire engine or an ambulance racing to the scene of an accident to save the victims in such a way as to kill several pedestrians along the way.[12] Finally, negligence takes account of the practicability of taking precautions (sometimes referred to as the burden of precautions or the cost of precautions) against the risk. If only comparatively small improvements in safety can be achieved by the expenditure of a large amount of resource, it may be reasonable not to undertake the precautions. This is meant as a measure of the objective reasonableness of the defendant's conduct. It does not mean that a defendant's lack of resources, e.g. in a public authority or a hospital, can justify a failure to take precautions that would otherwise be regarded as objectively reasonably required.

The factors taken into account by the courts in assessing negligence constitute a crude risk–benefit calculation. The process is crude simply because the court rarely has sufficient evidence to make a precise calculation of risks and benefits, and there are often a number of variables in play. It is sometimes said that the courts take a 'common-sense' approach, a phrase which may partly be a hangover from the days of jury trials (when juries were expected to apply the sense of the 'common man') but may also provide a 'comfort blanket' for the lack of precision in the exercise.

In the context of professional liability, and particularly medical negligence, much of the process of assessing benefits and risks is subsumed within the expert evidence. The phrase from McNair J's judgment that 'A doctor is not guilty of negligence if he has acted in accordance with a practice accepted as proper by a responsible body of medical men skilled in that particular art' has led to a tendency to rely on expert witnesses as a measure of what constitutes a 'responsible body of professional opinion'. One effect of the *Bolam* test is that even where experts for the claimant consider that the defendant's conduct was negligent if the evidence of the defendant's experts is to the contrary, and the court considers that this constitutes 'a responsible body of professional opinion', the claim will fail. The question of what constitutes a responsible body of professional opinion is, however, ultimately a matter for the court to decide. In *Bolitho* v. *City and Hackney Health Authority*[13] the House of Lords said that expert evidence must stand up to logical analysis:

> the court has to be satisfied that the exponents of the body of opinion relied upon can demonstrate that such opinion has a logical basis. In particular in cases involving, as they so often do, the weighing of risks against benefits, the judge before accepting a body of opinion as being responsible, reasonable or respectable, will need to be satisfied that, in forming their views, the experts have directed their minds to the question of comparative risks and benefits and have reached a defensible conclusion on the matter.

It will be rare, however, for the courts to reject the evidence of expert witnesses on the basis that their views do not stand up to logical analysis:

> In the vast majority of cases the fact that distinguished experts in the field are of a particular opinion will demonstrate the reasonableness of that opinion. In particular, where there are questions of assessment of the relative risks and benefits of adopting a particular medical practice, a reasonable view necessarily presupposes that the relative risks and benefits have been weighed by the experts in forming their opinions. But if, in a rare case, it can be demonstrated that the professional opinion is not capable of withstanding logical analysis, the judge is entitled to hold that the body of opinion is not reasonable or responsible.[14]

The relationship between litigation and medical practice

In theory, there should be a direct relationship between the safety of medical practice and litigation, a relationship that operates in two ways. First, the more unsafe medical practice is, the more adverse events will occur, and the more litigation should result. Conversely, the safer medical practice is, the fewer adverse events will occur, and the volume of litigation should reduce. Thus, there should be a link between improved risk management practices and less litigation. This is an intuitive judgment, but in practice the link is probably tenuous. The estimated annual number of adverse events in NHS hospitals in England is 850,000, of which about half are avoidable (Department of Health 2000; Vincent et al. 2001; Donaldson 2003). The number of avoidable adverse events caused by negligence is not known. The Harvard Medical Practice Study (Harvard Medical Practice Study 1990; Brennan et al. 1991; Leape et al. 1991; Localio et al. 1991) found that 1 per cent of hospital patients suffered injury as a result of negligence. If that figure is extrapolated to England and Wales, then about 85,000 hospital adverse events per annum are caused by negligence. The number of new claims for negligence being dealt with by the NHS Litigation Authority (NHSLA) is now around 7,000 per annum.[15] If there are 85,000 patients per annum who suffer injury as a result of negligence and only 7,000 claims (of which some 75 per cent may be unsuccessful[16]) then even if a risk management system was dramatically successful and reduced adverse events by, say, 50 per cent there would still be plenty of potential claimants, who currently do not make a claim, who could produce an increase in claims. Claims rates can change for a variety of reasons which have nothing at all to do with greater patient safety, or indeed despite improvements in patient safety.

The second aspect of the relationship between medical practice and litigation is based on the theory of general deterrence. The tort of negligence is often regarded as having the prime function of compensating the victims of negligence – its focus is on the claimant's right to a remedy once damage has occurred. But negligence should, in theory, also have the capacity to deter the wrongful conduct of the defendant through the threat of imposing liability. Deterrence is generally regarded as having a powerful role in the criminal law, but there are areas of the civil law that also have a deterrent function (the law of defamation is perhaps a classic example). The difficulty with the tort of negligence as a deterrent of wrongful conduct (or an 'incentive' to safer conduct) is twofold. First, in practice, the link between the 'actor' whose conduct is characterized as negligent and the 'penalty' imposed (in the form of an award of damages to the claimant) is tenuous. In the private sector the defendant is usually insured and therefore does not pay the damages himself, and the negligent actor is often an employee for whose negligence an employer is held vicariously liable. In theory, an insurance company, having paid the claimant's damages by virtue of the defendant's liability insurance policy, has the right to seek an indemnity from the defendant's negligent employee. In practice, as a result of a 'gentleman's agreement' with the government, this right (often practically worthless, in any event) is not enforced by the insurance industry, unless there is evidence of wilful misconduct or fraud by the employee. In the NHS, apart from claims against general practitioners,[17] again it is not the negligent health professional who pays the claimant's damages. And although the NHS Trust has an incentive to adopt the NHS Litigation Authority risk management standards in order to receive a discount on its contribution to the Clinical Negligence Scheme for Trusts (CNST), as with liability insurance, there is no direct link between the negligent defendant and the body paying compensation. In theory, the potential for disciplinary action against an errant doctor or health professional should have some deterrent effect on professional conduct, though it would be rare for a single instance of negligence to lead to disciplinary action, e.g. by the General Medical Council. The error would have to be very serious.

The second, and probably more significant, flaw in the theory of deterrence is the nature of the conduct that has to be deterred and the guidance that the law can give. Many cases of negligence probably consist of inadvertence to the dangerous consequences of the defendant's conduct. If in fact the health professional does not foresee the danger, even though he ought reasonably to have foreseen it, he cannot take precautions against it. Moreover, a general exhortation to 'be careful' is not specific enough to give useful guidance as to how people should behave, and the courts must inevitably rule on whether the defendant has been sufficiently careful after the event.

Defensive medicine

The aspect of the relationship between litigation and medical practice that tends to receive the greatest attention, at least in the medical press, is 'defensive medicine'.

This is the argument that, in response to the threat of litigation, doctors practise defensively, which involves undertaking procedures which are not medically justified for the patient's benefit but are designed to protect the doctor from a claim for negligence. The most commonly cited examples are unnecessary diagnostic tests, such as X-rays, and unnecessary Caesarian section deliveries. Given the nature of the *Bolam* test, however, these claims do not make a great deal of sense, because a reasonable doctor would not undertake an *unnecessary* procedure and so a doctor cannot avoid a finding of negligence by performing one; and to the extent that the procedure carries some inherent risk, the practitioner acting in this way may increase the chances of being sued. Moreover, there is little clear understanding within the medical profession of what 'defensive medicine' means.[18] 'Defensive' may mean simply treating patients conservatively or even 'more carefully', and this begs the question whether that treatment option is medically justified in the patient's interests. Uncertainty as to the optimal level of care leads to economic inefficiency in the operation of liability rules (Fenn et al. 2004).

The concept of defensive medicine essentially involves a judgment that imposing liability for negligence will tend to 'over-deter' potential defendants, damaging the service in question, rather than contributing to an improvement in standards of conduct. Logically, the same argument would apply to any defendant who is held accountable in the tort of negligence, but no one suggests that imposing a duty to exercise reasonable care on, say, motorists makes them drive *too* carefully. Sometimes the problem is expressed in terms of potential defendants approaching their professional responsibilities in a 'defensive frame of mind', the assumption being that this is a negative consequence. To an objective observer, however, the defendant professional's frame of mind is irrelevant, provided that objectively his/her conduct conforms to the standard of reasonable care. The 'frame of mind' with which any professional person approaches the tasks to be carried out is so subjective as to be almost meaningless. What is 'defensive' for one may well be regarded as good practice by another. What counts is whether *objectively* the professional is exercising reasonable standards of professional conduct. Moreover, the fact that doctors invoke the concept of defensive medicine suggests that doctors do respond to the threat of liability, that legal rules do have a deterrent effect.

The argument that the deterrent effect of liability rules is harmful to the practice of medicine (and therefore the interests of patients) is inherently contradictory. It makes no sense to argue that liability rules over-deter defendants, changing good practice into bad practice, if they do not also have some deterrent effect on poor practice, thereby improving patient safety.

Implications of the law's approach for patient safety

Lawyers act as the pathologists of adverse events, but their focus is strictly limited to the process of attributing legal responsibility for the consequences of, usually, a single adverse event. It is not their role to identify systemic problems in a service, though their experience of dealing with claims may give them some insight into this. The cases that lawyers see are probably not entirely representative of the range of adverse events – they tend to be limited to those incidents that cause the greatest damage or loss, which are more likely to be worth litigating – though there are some patterns that emerge (see Chapter 4 of Jones 2003). Very occasionally, there may be a specific response by the NHS to specific incidents, such as the changes introduced following the scandal of organ retention at Alder Hey hospital, but generally the law is very limited in terms of its ability to produce improvements in safety practice as a response to a single incident. One reason for this is that, although it is theoretically possible to litigate an instance of negligence on the basis that harm to the patient arose from an error in the organization of healthcare delivery, it is difficult to prove that the organization itself was at fault, particularly where the practice in question is commonly adopted by other hospitals. For example, it may be standard practice for NHS hospitals to leave inadequately supervised, and inexperienced, staff at the front line of healthcare delivery, partly through lack of resources and partly as a means of giving 'hands-on training'. It would be difficult for a judge to condemn as negligent a practice widely adopted in the NHS, even if it is recognized that this increases the risk of harm to patients, because it would probably have major financial, and possibly political, implications for the NHS. It is far easier for a judge to apply the objective standard of the *Bolam* test, where inexperience is not a defence, to conclude that the individual doctor or nurse at the end of the chain of responsibility was negligent, and then hold the NHS Trust vicariously liable for that individual negligent mistake. Claimants' lawyers recognize this and frame claims accordingly.

Ironically, perhaps, the main contribution to patient safety that litigation has made is the rise in the annual cost of litigation to the NHS. The actual cost is around £450 million per annum[19] (not the several billions that National Audit Office reports as provisions in the NHS account). The NHS (England) Summarised Accounts 2002–2003[20] made 'provisions' for claims amounting to £5.89 billion. This is a figure which takes account of all known claims, and all future claims which could give rise to liability for clinical negligence, including estimates for incurred but not reported claims (i.e. for incidents where patients may have suffered injury but have not yet made a claim). At 31 March 2004, the NHS Litigation Authority estimated that it had potential clinical negligence liabilities of £7.78 billion. The estimates have changed because the 'discount rate' set by the government was changed on 1 April 2003 from 6 per cent to 3.5 per cent, not because of any increase in claims rates.[21] These estimates give a highly misleading picture of the financial position, since: (1) they are based on assumptions about the success rates of claimants which are unlikely to be achieved in practice; (2) they give the impression that the cost of claims is running at a much higher level than £440 to £450 million per annum (the equivalent in the context of the overall NHS budget would be to add up the salary costs of all staff working in the NHS over, say, the next 10 or 15 years, and say that the resulting figure of several hundred (or thousand) billion of pounds represents the real cost of running the NHS – it is like comparing the monthly cost of paying a mortgage with the outstanding indebtedness represented by the mortgage itself).

It may be cynical to suggest that it is this bottom line that has provided the incentive for the NHS as a whole to take risk management seriously, but there is little evidence that health professionals, despite the ethical injunction to 'do no harm', took patient safety seriously before litigation began to 'take off' in the 1980s. Indeed, the first reaction of the medical profession to the effects of increased litigation in the

1980s (increased subscription rates to the defence organizations) was to blame others (greedy lawyers, ungrateful patients, gullible judges, and the naïve Legal Aid Board (Jones 1987)) rather than admit that maybe health care was the problem rather than the victim. Thus, what litigation in general has achieved is to create the environment in which the NHS has had to take risk management and patient safety seriously. The NHSLA offers reduced subscription rates to CNST for NHS Trusts that meet its risk management standards, on the assumption that there is a correlation between taking patient safety seriously and reducing the number of claims for negligence. Though as Fenn et al. (2004) point out, these discounts are a reflection of processes rather than outcomes. It is simply assumed that improved risk-management processes result in better outcomes in terms of reduced adverse events and/or claims. There is no empirical evidence, however, establishing a direct link between improved patient safety and reduced litigation costs.[22] Nonetheless, it is clear that the overall cost of claims is a significant driver of the medico-political agenda. For example, the Department of Health has stated that birth-related brain damage (including cerebral palsy) in England accounted for just over 5 per cent of all cases of medical litigation in which damages were paid, but 60 per cent of all expenditure on medical litigation. As a consequence, recommendations for reform made in *Making Amends* targeted brain-damaged baby cases for special compensation arrangements outside the legal system.[23]

Probably the central issue in terms of the implications for patient safety of the legal perspective is whether the law really does have a deterrent effect on careless practice which enhances patient safety. In theory, there should be a correlation between litigation levels and patient safety, but the uncertainties involved in determining what is an appropriate level of care are compounded by the *Bolam* test which allows for multiple standards of 'responsible professional practice'. This means that the law adopts the lowest common denominator in terms of what is considered to be appropriate medical practice, rather than searching for the optimal level of care as a relevant standard. It is, arguably, the existence of the litigation process, and the overall cost to the NHS of dealing with the consequences of negligently inflicted injuries, that have produced the greatest spur to improved patient safety, but the *process* of identifying what constitutes 'safe' or appropriate practice falls largely beyond the scope of the legal system. The courts do not presume to tell doctors how they should practise medicine, except in the limited number of cases where a particular practice seems to be so obviously contrary to an intuitive risk–benefit calculation that it cannot pass muster as withstanding logical analysis. Finally, it may be argued that there could be lessons for patient safety to be taken from claims analysis. On the other hand, the fairly random nature of claims may prevent truly systematic analysis of the causes of error.

Notes

1   Comments on the law refer to the law of England and Wales. Scotland has a different jurisdiction, though the principles of the law of negligence are virtually the same.

2   [1957] 2 All ER 118, 121.

3 [1957] 2 All ER 118, 122.

4 *Glasgow Corporation v Muir* [1943] AC 448, 457.

5 *Nettleship v Weston* [1971] 2 QB 691, 698, 710 – learner driver held to the same standard of competence as an experienced driver; *Jones v Manchester Corporation* [1952] QB 852, 871 – inexperienced anaesthetist liable for accidentally overdosing, and killing, the patient: 'Errors due to inexperience or lack of supervision are no defence as against the injured person.' The inexperienced professional can avoid liability by having his/her work checked by a more senior colleague: *Wilsher v Essex Area Health Authority* [1987] QB 730.

6 *Wilsher v Essex Area Health Authority* [1987] QB 730, 747, *per* Mustill LJ.

7 A 'tort' (from the French 'wrong') is simply a civil wrong giving rise to a claim for damages that is not based on breach of contract. There are various torts, including negligence, nuisance, trespass, defamation, and so on.

8 *Roe v Minister of Health* [1954] 2 QB 66 – defendants not liable for patient's paralysis caused by contamination of the anaesthetic by an unforeseen mechanism.

9 *Bolton v Stone* [1951] AC 850.

10 *Paris v Stepney Borough Council* [1951] AC 367.

11 *Watt v Hertfordshire County Council* [1954] 1 WLR 835.

12 So it can be negligence for the driver of a fire engine or ambulance to ignore a red traffic-light, even in an emergency: *Ward v London County Council* [1938] 2 All ER 341; *Griffin v Mersey Regional Ambulance* [1998] PIQR P34.

13 [1998] AC 232, 241–242.

14 [1998] AC 232, 243.

15 In 2002–3 there were 6,797 new claims received (according to Donaldson (2003), p. 58, para. 32), though the NHS Litigation Authority states that the number was 7,798 new claims received (*NHSLA Fact Sheet* No. 3, August 2004). The figure for 2003–4 fell to 6,251 new claims (*NHSLA Fact Sheet* No. 3, August 2004) [the *Fact Sheets* are available at www.nhsla.com].

16 Note that this depends upon how the figures are calculated, and varies with the source. National Audit Office (2001), p. 32 stated that for clinical negligence claims funded by legal aid (which is more than 90 per cent of all such claims) for 1999–2000 only 24 per cent of claimants were successful. However, the NHSLA suggests that, as at 31 March 2004, the success rate for claimants is about 45 per cent: *NHSLA Fact Sheet* No. 3 (August 2004).

17 The position of general practitioners is complicated by the fact that some may be employees (e.g. of a Primary Care Trust), though most are, in effect, self-employed. Self-employed general practitioners can obtain indemnity against negligence claims through subscription to a defence organization, usually the Medical Defence Union or the Medical Protection Society. The National Health Service (General Medical Services Contracts) Regulations 2004 (S.I. 2004 No. 291) Sch. 6, para. 122 and the National Health Service (Personal Medical Services Agreements) Regulations 2004 (S.I. 2004 No. 627) Sch. 5, para. 113 make professional indemnity insurance compulsory for general practitioners.

18 See Jones and Morris (1989), cf. Tribe and Korgaonkar (1991); Summerton (1995).

19 The NHS Litigation Authority has reported that it actually paid out £446.2 million in 2002–2003 and £442.5 million in 2003–2004: *NHSLA Fact Sheet*, No. 2, August 2004.
20 Available at www.nao.gov.uk
21 *NHSLA Fact Sheet*, No. 2, August 2004.
22 Fenn et al. (2004) at 1:279 report that hospitals that had a high excess level for contributions to CNST had a reduced frequency of claims. In other words, where the organization had a direct financial interest in meeting the cost of claims it took steps to reduce claims frequency. From 1 April 2002, excesses have been reduced to zero for all NHS Trusts and all claims are now managed directly by the NHSLA.
23 Donaldson (2003), p. 47, para. 43.

Box 6.1 Key points

- The *Bolam* test for negligence sets an objective standard of reasonable care, which is normally measured by reference to the relevant professional standards.
- In assessing relevant professional standards, through the evidence of expert witnesses, the court will enquire whether the views expressed stand up to logical analysis.
- This involves undertaking a broad risk–benefit analysis of the events in question.
- The law always views matters in retrospect, though negligence is measured by reference to reasonable *foresight* at the time of the events in question.
- In theory, the risk of liability for negligence should provide a deterrent to unsafe conduct, but in practice the deterrent effect is significantly diluted.
- The concept of 'defensive medicine' involves an assertion that liability for negligence over-deters potential defendants, producing potentially harmful consequences for patients, but this is conceptually incoherent.
- The legal system is good at providing a forensic investigation into what went wrong in an individual case, and allocating responsibility for that, but is not good at identifying organizational issues which hamper patient safety.
- There is an assumption that improved patient safety will reduce the levels of (and therefore the cost of) litigation but, although intuitively this assumption seems reasonable, there is no empirical evidence indicating a direct link between safety standards and levels of litigation.

References

Brennan, T.A., Leape, L.L., Laird, N.M., Hebert, L., Localio, A.R., Lawthers, A.G., Newhouse, J.P., Weiler, P.C. and Hiatt, H.H. (1991) Incidence of adverse events and negligence in hospitalized patients: Results of the Harvard Medical Practice Study, *New England Journal of Medicine*, 325 (Feb 7): 370–6.
Department of Health (2000) *An Organization with a Memory*. London: The Stationery Office.
Donaldson, L. (2003) *Making Amends: A Consultation Paper Setting out Proposals for Reforming the Approach to Clinical Negligence in the NHS*. London: The Stationery Office.

Fenn, P., Gray, A. and Rickman, N. (2004) The economics of clinical negligence reform in England, *The Economic Journal*, 114: F272, at F275–F276.

Harvard Medical Practice Study (1990) *Patients, Doctors and Lawyers: Medical Injury, Malpractice Litigation and Patient Compensation in New York*. Boston, MA: Harvard College.

Jones, M.A. (1987) The rising cost of medical malpractice, *Professional Negligence*, 3(2): 43–6.

Jones, M.A. (2003) *Medical Negligence*. 3rd edn. London: Sweet and Maxwell.

Jones, M.A. and Morris, A.E. (1989) Defensive medicine: myths and facts, *Journal of the Medical Defence Union*, 5(40).

Leape, L.L., Brennan, T.A., Laird, N., Lawthers, A.G., Localio, A.R., Barnes, B.A., Hebert, L., Newhouse, J.P., Weiler, P.C. and Hiatt, H. (1991) The nature of adverse events in hospitalized patients: Results of the Harvard Medical Practice Study II, *New England Journal of Medicine*, 325 (Feb 7): 377–84.

Localio, A.R, Lawthers, A.G., Brennan, T.A., Laird, N.M., Hebert, L.E., Peterson, L.M., Newhouse, J.P., Weiler, P.C. and Hiatt, H.H. (1991) Relation between malpractice claims and adverse events due to negligence: Results of the Harvard Medical Practice Study III, *New England Journal of Medicine*, 325 (Feb 7): 245–51.

National Audit Office (2001) *Handling Clinical Negligence Claims in England*, London: The Stationery Office.

Summerton, N. (1995) Positive and negative factors in defensive medicine: a questionnaire study of general practitioners, *British Medical Journal*, 310: 27–9.

Tribe, D. and Korgaonkar, G. (1991) The impact of litigation on patient care: an enquiry into defensive medical practice, *Professional Negligence* 7(2): 6.

Vincent, C., Neale, G. et al. (2001) Adverse events in British hospitals: preliminary retrospective record review, *British Medical Journal*, 322: 517–19.

PART 2
Approaches to evaluating
patient safety

7

Developing and using taxonomies of errors

Sue Dovey, John Hickner and Bob Phillips

'Please bring me the red dress.'

'Do you mean the one with the white polka dots?'

What is the dress? Is it a red dress, or is it a white polka dot dress? Dr Michael Ghiselin, noted biologist and taxonomist, used this example to set the stage for a discussion of the ambiguities inherent in formal systems of classification, or taxonomies. A taxonomy is a classification system for ordering things into groups based on their similarity. The characteristics of the objects, events or phenomena that one uses to classify them, however, are always somewhat arbitrary.

Classifying objects can be difficult, but classifying events is even more so. Consider the following real patient safety event report:

> The husband of a 74-year-old patient called in with complaints that she had had diarrhea, with occasional incontinence. She has dementia and Parkinson's, and it seemed as if the diarrhea and incontinence could be related to these chronic problems, without much chance of satisfactory resolution. A stool sample was dropped off for analysis at the clinic and was negative for everything but blood. The results sat in a stack of papers for a week, until the husband called in saying she was weak and having black stools. She came in for a hemo-globin, which was found to be critically low. She was admitted to the hospital, transfused, and scoped. She was found to have stomach ulcers from the arthritis medication she had taken for a decade. The patient's husband thinks that she had a small stroke during the episode, the symptoms of which have now resolved. She spent the weekend in the hospital. I have a chaotic work environ-ment and am way behind on paperwork. My piles of thing to do grow larger every day.

> (Reporter – physician)

Under what rubric shall we classify this event? Is it a medication event, a communica-tion event, a geriatric event? If patient safety events – or incidents – must be classified in mutually exclusive categories, what type of event is this? It depends on the structure of the taxonomy.

In this chapter we will first discuss principles of classification and how these principles apply to patient safety taxonomies. Then we will discuss the classification of medical errors, also called patient safety events/incidents. We will summarize existing approaches to the reporting and classification of medical errors, providing examples of how patient safety taxonomies are useful to direct improvement efforts to areas in which they are most needed. We will conclude with comments about the future of patient safety taxonomy and suggestions for users and researchers.

General principles of classification and their application to patient safety

Careful thought about the purpose of a taxonomy (classification system) guided by theory and practical experience is necessary to develop a functional taxonomy. There is a delicate interplay between the theoretical framework of a body of knowledge and the classification system used to codify that knowledge. Knowledge, understanding, and theory change over time; sometimes advanced by intellectual insights (theory development) and sometimes by empirical discoveries. Science is an iterative process that uses inductive and deductive reasoning; specific findings to general rules; general rules applied to specific findings. The role of classification systems is to organize and display specific, empirical findings in ways that enhance understanding. The periodic table, for example, was originally constructed to represent 'families' of elements with similar chemical properties – not as an expression of theory. However, understanding the theoretical framework underlying a classification system is necessary to fully comprehend the data. The periodic table means a great deal more to those who know what protons, neutrons and electrons are. Taxonomies are powerful political and social tools as well, and they reflect prevailing societal beliefs. As evidence, one need only recall that homosexuality was an abnormal psychiatric diagnosis in previous versions of medical classifications.

An ideal classification system should have mutually exclusive categories and be exhaustive. That is, an event or object may not be located in more than one place in the classification system, and all events of the type being classified must fit somewhere. A library book, for example, can have only one identification number in the Dewey decimal system and can occupy only one spot on the shelves, and all books can be assigned an identification number. But many phenomena are multi-dimensional, especially patient safety events such as the event described above. Therefore, patient safety classification systems must be multi-dimensional in order to provide comprehensive summaries of events. The advent of computerized databases has made multi-axial classification systems easier to create and use for analyses. One can attach many names or codes to a given object or event. When one wishes to retrieve all the objects that have similar characteristics, it is as simple as pressing a button. The difficulty with the database approach, if not developed with appropriate conceptual models, is that it may not provide a hierarchy of objects or events that are related in some important ways. Hierarchical organization of categories facilitates understanding of similarities and differences. Modern classification systems can take advantage of both approaches.

In developing a classification system, one may start either with a conceptual framework or with data. For example, one might ask a pharmacist to list everything that might go wrong in medication prescribing or one could ask the pharmacist to report all the errors she observes during the next month. Either approach relies on close familiarity with the area of interest. The advantage of a theory-driven approach is that the categories are likely to be related in important and logical ways from the beginning. The advantage of the empirical, data-driven approach is that one is not constrained by the initial categories or the taxonomists' biases. In reality, classification systems evolve as one moves from data to theory and back to data again, as with any scientific process.

Taxonomists must ask themselves four questions before they begin their work. What do we want to classify? What kind of thing is it? Why do we want to classify it? What sort of classification is appropriate? Although the answer to 'What do we want to classify?' might appear straightforward, let us again consider the red dress. What is a dress? Is it a one-piece garment worn by women that covers the body? Is a tunic, then, a dress? Is a sari a dress? What about a kimono? Different classifiers might have different answers to these questions, and even expert dressmakers might not agree. Usually it is possible to agree on including or excluding objects that fit centrally or not at all into a classification scheme. Around the boundaries classification becomes much more difficult. We see this problem appearing in patient safety taxonomies. Do we include all adverse events regardless of cause or only those due to error? Does one include only errors that resulted in harm to a patient? What constitutes harm? The Institute of Medicine definition of medical errors includes errors of commission and errors of omission. Does this mean that failure to perform a recommended screening test for cancer is a medical error? If so, are all quality-related events and non-events medical errors? Furthermore, are we speaking about medical errors or healthcare errors? Whose actions, then, shall we include? If a patient does not adhere to a dietary regimen, is that an error? Or, is the patient simply exercising her autonomy? A broad definition of medical errors has the advantage of including important 'latent errors' of healthcare policy and organization but has the disadvantage of distracting the patient safety conversation from the most urgent goal – avoiding actively harming people from medical interventions. The importance of boundaries cannot be overstated. Objects or events that do not fit into the taxonomy become invisible.

What kind of thing is it? Most generally, a dress is a garment. But a dress may also be a fashion statement, a way to attract attention, or a ceremonial symbol. When considering medical errors, do we mean discrete mistakes by individuals, or shall we include systems problems and organizational problems? Errors that harm patients are frequently the result of a series of errors that can be due to human error, systems design flaws, and organizational problems; hence the terminology 'patient safety event'. Shall we seek, then, to classify individual errors or events? The correct answer is 'it depends'. Because most of the taxonomies of patient safety have been developed in association with event reporting, patient safety taxonomies, in reality, classify events that pose a threat to patients' safety rather than the individual errors that combine to form the event. It is important to note that not all safety events result in harm. There is value in studying 'near misses' as well because they can reveal what went right as well as what went wrong.

Why do we want to classify it? The purpose of a taxonomy is to organize knowledge to facilitate understanding. Taxonomies are fundamental to knowledge organization and communication. They provide a framework for understanding new discoveries. They facilitate critical thinking. They allow comparison and conversation between those interested in a particular field of human endeavour. Taxonomies include definitions of words and rules of classification that facilitate meaningful discussion and communication. Classification relates the general to the specific, 'kinds' to 'instances'. The most useful classification systems also address the issues of aetiology, cause and effect. Therefore, the fundamental characteristics or 'dimensions' of the things being classified that one selects for a taxonomy are crucial.

The purpose of patient safety taxonomies should be to facilitate understanding of threats to safety in a way that informs efforts to reduce harm. Patient safety taxonomies must be useful to a variety of users, including policy-makers, healthcare administrators, quality managers, healthcare personnel including practitioners and staff, and safety researchers. A patient safety taxonomy's value should be judged on how well it organizes data to create knowledge and understanding to inform improvement. A good patient safety taxonomy helps to identify and clarify the safety issues in medicine and it provides a foundation for resolving those problems. A good taxonomy serves as the basis for action.

What sort of classification system is appropriate? Biologists and zoologists decided some time ago that plants and animals ought to be classified according to their phylogeny, their evolutionary origin. Physicists have developed an elegant taxonomy for the elements of matter, the periodic table. A variety of taxonomies and nomenclatures exist for defining classifying medical terms and procedures. These include the International Classification of Disease (ICD), Read Codes, and International Classification of Primary Care (ICPC) for diagnoses; Current Procedural Terminology (CPT) for procedures, and nomenclatures such as the Systemized Nomenclature of Human and Veterinary Medicine, Clinical Terms (SNOMED-CT) for categorizing medical phenomena, and Logical Observation Identifiers Names and Codes (LOINC) for describing and coding laboratory and related data. These are useful for classifying patient safety events, but none were designed as comprehensive classification systems for medical errors or adverse events. All of these taxonomies are dynamic, changing to accommodate new discoveries. With the sequencing of the human genome, these medical classification systems and nomenclatures are likely to change radically.

Patient safety taxonomies

With the increased focus on patient safety in the twenty-first century that was accelerated by the 1999 Institute of Medicine publication, *To Err is Human* (Institute of Medicine 1999), hundreds of adverse event reporting systems and patient safety taxonomies have sprung up. An indication of the intensity of interest in patient safety taxonomy is the 60,300 hits we received on *Google* under 'patient safety taxonomy' in January 2005. Most existing patient safety taxonomies are home-grown classification systems used by hospitals and healthcare organizations to organize their adverse event reports. At least half of the states in the USA have mandatory reporting requirements for serious adverse events that occur in hospital, and each of these states uses a different classification system. While local, and regional taxonomies are useful for regulation and local improvement, it is not possible to compare data from different sites because of the lack of standard terminology and categories. Some patient safety taxonomies are specific to certain specialties, such as anaesthesia, neonatology, pediatrics, or general practice. The ICD-9/10 CM External Cause and Injury Codes (E-Codes) is the classification system used most frequently in US hospitals for classifying adverse events. Only a handful of taxonomies have tackled the larger issues of national and international standardization, allowing comparisons of patient safety events more universally across the continuum of care.

Like the periodic table, most existing patient safety taxonomies started with *observations* of events that visibly (usually physically) harmed patients but unlike most other scientific taxonomies, 'families' of events in patient safety taxonomies tend to be defined not by their aetiology, but by their ultimate outcome. Theory has come later and is currently in rapid development, paralleling the rapid recent accumulation of safety event descriptions. Patient safety taxonomies must start with a clear understanding of their purpose. Most often this purpose has been to provide information to help staff in hospitals and primary care clinics provide care that helps, rather than harms, patients. To provide rich enough descriptions to develop interventions, patient safety taxonomies need to be multi-dimensional. Different developers have arrived at a variety of conclusions regarding the number and types of major domains (axes) to include in a patient safety taxonomy. At a minimum, however, the taxonomy must include domains to describe the context of the event (who, what, when, where) and presumed underlying causes of the event (why). Here, we describe four general patient safety taxonomies and two primary care taxonomies, outlining unique features of each.

The Australian Incident Monitoring System (AIMS) and the General Occurrence Classification (GOC)

The first attempt to develop a comprehensive patient safety taxonomy started in Australia. In 1987 William Runciman and his colleagues launched the Australian Incident Monitoring System (AIMS) to monitor anaesthesia mishaps (Runciman 2002). In the mid-1990s as AIMS expanded to encompass 'things that go wrong' throughout the healthcare system, AIMS researchers developed the Generic Occurrence Classification (GOC) for patient safety events (Runciman et al. 1998). They discovered that existing classifications such as the Read Codes or ICD-9 E Codes were insufficient to describe what goes wrong in health care. To guide development of the GOC, Runciman and colleagues outlined a comprehensive model for understanding patient safety events called the Generic Reference Model (Figure 7.1) that has three major categories: contributing factors and hazards, descriptors of the incident, and outcomes and consequences. This is based on the widely used 'Reason' model of complex systems failure. Using 1,000 reports of patient safety incidents in teaching hospitals, he classified the main features of these reports into 'natural categories' using a process called 'natural mapping' (Norman 1998). A natural category is a descriptor that is brief, easily and commonly understood which captures the essence of an event and is not constrained by being restricted to any class. Natural mapping refers to connecting groups of natural categories in an intuitively reasonable way.

APSF Generic Reference Model – based on
Reason's model of complex system failure

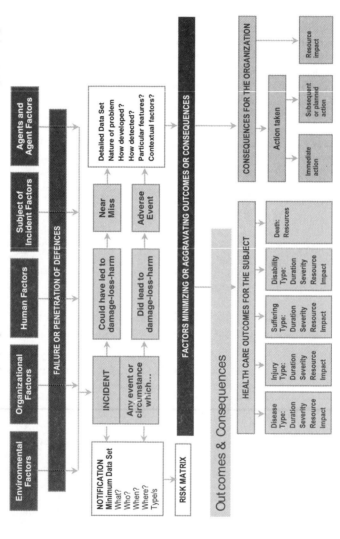

Figure 7.1 The Generic Reference Model of the Australian Incident Monitoring System
Source: Reprinted with permission of W. Runciman and the Australian Patient Safety Foundation

The GOC is not, strictly speaking, a taxonomy but rather a huge computerized branching database that elegantly organizes salient and important elements of an incident report in a way that preserves the narrative description yet allows complex analyses of relationships among many variables. One begins coding an event into the system by starting with the Health Incident Type. The data entry operator follows the computer tree branches to the last branch or as far as data allow. It is not possible to display this complex database on paper; only segments of the trees, as it has over 1.5 million permutations. For less serious events, an abridged form can be used. Domain-specific computer programs that use the same structure as the GOC are being developed that will simplify data entry for specific healthcare venues such as nursing homes and general practice. This system is a powerful engine for analysis of patient safety issues but requires considerable training to enter data properly. AIMS is perhaps unique in that it is designed to receive reports from a wide variety of sources including incident monitoring, medical record review, death certificates, hospital discharges, surveys of general practice, patient complaints, medico-legal investigations, coroner investigations, results of other enquires and investigators and even literature searches.

The Medical Event Reporting System (MERS)

In the mid-1990s Hal Kaplan and colleagues at the University of Texas Southwestern in Dallas developed an incident monitoring system for transfusion medicine, MERS-TM. At Columbia University in New York, he and his team have since expanded this system to capture events from all healthcare domains and settings. MERS-TH (Medical Event Reporting System – Total HealthSystem) is a web-based approach designed to collect, classify, analyse and monitor events that could potentially compromise patient safety. It provides the opportunity to study events and their associated causes to facilitate the development of corrective actions and process improvement efforts that will reduce future risk of harm.

The MERS-TH 'process' includes the following steps: Detection, Selection, Investigation, Description and Classification, Computation, and Interpretation. Each step involves a standardized process and associated tools. Coding, using the system's unique event and root cause taxonomies, takes place during Description and Classification and is heavily relied upon for Computation and Interpretation strategies. The taxonomy was specifically developed to capture reports of actual events (with and without associated harm), near-miss events, 'dangerous' situations, and clinical adverse events. In contrast to Runciman's very empirical method of getting started, Kaplan chose to ground his root cause taxonomy in general safety theory, with the goal of assigning causal codes to each 'branch' of an event. He reasoned that a safety taxonomy should, above all, produce understanding of causation as a first step in understanding and avoiding similar mishaps in the future. Kaplan and van der Schaaf adapted an existing causal classification model originally developed for safety event reporting in the chemical industry (Van der Schaaf 1992). The Eindhoven Classification Model for Medical Domain has three main causal categories: latent errors (technical and organizational), active errors (human), and other (patient-related and unclassifiable). These categories are consistent with the theoretical frameworks of Reason and Rasmussen (Rasmussen 1987; Reason 1990).

In addition to the causal codes that are assigned to root causes that led up to the mishap, MERS includes many contextual variables for comparative analyses that were developed after reviewing other patient safety systems, which for the most part were domain-specific. Information is shared by the reporter using a computerized, standardized approach (searchable fields, drop-down lists), and both the 'discovery' situation and the 'occurrence' situation of each event are coded using a four-tiered taxonomy model: Service, Event Type (broad category), Event Description (specific event), and Contributing Factor(s). If a root cause analysis is performed (risk analysis and search tools are provided to assist in decision-making), multiple chronological 'layers' of the chain of occurrences that led up to the event are coded. Initially, this taxonomy was tested using a retrospective sampling of event reports. It was then piloted in limited hospital units, followed by a full rollout throughout both hospital and ambulatory care settings. Like AIMS, MERS is not, strictly speaking, a taxonomy, but rather a powerful structured relational computer database and tool for causal analyses. It requires a skilled systems operator to perform the coding and root cause analysis.

The National Reporting and Learning System (NRLS)

Development of the National Patient Safety Agency (NPSA) taxonomy started in 2002 with an examination of other patient safety-related classifications used in the UK. From this analysis the most suitable classification was chosen and piloted, but due to its acute sector focus the Agency decided to develop its own taxonomy to cover the needs of all service sectors. Reference groups for nine service areas (acute, ambulance, dentistry, general practice, optometry, mental health, learning disabilities, pharmacy and primary care) were established. These groups were made up of internal NPSA staff, service representatives, the Royal Colleges and healthcare associated charities. The taxonomy then developed iteratively and once the groups were comfortable with its structure and nomenclature it was re-piloted.

A web-enabled electronic eForm was developed to allow reporters to submit live patient safety-related data to the NPSA. During this phase some 12,000 reports were submitted and analysed by NPSA statisticians. In addition to this empirical analysis, anecdotal evidence on the quality and usability of the taxonomy was gathered from user feedback and usability studies. To work through all of these inputs, a series of intensive workshops were held, bringing together NPSA staff and external experts representing all the service areas, with the aim to rationalize and harmonize the taxonomy. The patient safety incident type taxonomy was a key focus area during these workshops. Prior to the workshop, each service area had a distinct patient safety incident categorization that meant there were around 300 incident types in total. With such a categorization, statistical cross-service comparative analysis was almost impossible. It was therefore clear that for meaningful information to be obtained from the system, the NPSA needed to rationalize and standardize the taxonomy.

To achieve this harmonization, participants from different service areas were mixed together to encourage sharing of knowledge and experience. A series of card-sorting workshops took place to agree on the classification, which led to a standardized terminology to describe incident types and a cross-service incident classification

(Table 7.1). This has established an excellent basis from which to compile cross-service statistical reports that will highlight issues, themes and national trends worthy of further investigation.

The JCAHO Patient Safety Event Taxonomy (PSET)

The Joint Commission on Accreditation of Hospitals and Healthcare Organizations (JCAHO) is the largest independent accrediting agency for medical organizations in the United States. In 2003–4 a team of researchers from JCAHO took a different approach to developing a taxonomy. The investigators not only incorporated the best features of several existing taxonomies, but also utilized an extensive review of the literature and the Joint Commission's Sentinel Event Database to populate taxonomy elements (Chang et al. 2005). They sought to 'identify similarities and gaps in the terminology and classifications to create a multidimensional taxonomy that encompasses diverse health care settings and incident reporting systems' (Chang et al. 2005). The JCAHO Patient Safety Event Taxonomy has five primary classification domains: impact, type, domain, cause, and prevention and mitigation (Table 7.2). Impact is the outcome or effects of medical error and systems failure, commonly

Table 7.1 Domains and primary categories of the NPSA patient safety taxonomy

Incident types	Contributory factors	Harm
Access, admission, transfer, discharge	Organization and strategic working conditions	No harm
Clinical assessment (incl. diagnosis, tests, assessments)	Team and social task factors	Impact prevented
Consent, communication, confidentiality	Patient factors	Impact not prevented
Disruptive, aggressive behaviour	Communication	Low
Documentation (including records, identification)	Education and training	Moderate
Infection control	Medication	Severe
Implementation and ongoing monitoring/review	Equipment and resources	Death
Infrastructure (including staffing, facilities, environment)		
Medical device, equipment		
Medication		
Patient abuse		
Patient accident		
Self-harming behaviour		
Treatment, procedure		
Other		

In addition to incident type, contributory factors and harm, data is gathered regarding the service area, location, staff type, specialty, medications and devices involved in the incident.

Table 7.2 Domains and primary categories of the JCAHO taxonomy

Impact	Type	Domain	Cause	Prevention and mitigation
medical	communication	setting	systems	universal
psychological	patient management	staff	(structure and	selective
physical	clinical performance	patient	process)	indicated
non-medical		target	technical	
legal			organizational	
social			human	
economic				

referred to as harm to the patient. Type is the implied or visible processes that were faulty or failed. Domain is the characteristics of the setting in which an incident occurred and the type of individuals involved. Cause is the factors and agents that led to an incident. Prevention and mitigation are the measures taken or proposed to reduce incidence and effects of adverse occurrences.

A preliminary test of the alpha version taxonomy conducted at one hospital with an active incident reporting system (Stanford's ICUsrs) demonstrated acceptable correlation between its coded categories (n = 111) and the categorized data requirements of the system. Thirteen (12 per cent) categories were identical, 42 (38 per cent) were synonymous, 45 (41 per cent) were related, and 6 (5 per cent) had to be extrapolated. Five (4 per cent) categories were unmatched – date and time of incident, patient or family dissatisfaction, and two patient identifiers – and were therefore omitted from the taxonomy.

Dimensions of Medical Outcomes (DMO)

The Dimensions of Medical Outcomes (DMO) taxonomy is designed to provide a detailed description of the processes and individuals involved in unsatisfactory patient outcomes, including events with and without identified errors, across all locations of medical care. The DMO taxonomy was developed using a theoretical model based on error processes as opposed to clinical domains. In the DMO framework, causation codes are considered within the general domain of a system, individual or institutional process. The original taxonomy was then iteratively enhanced and refined through coding of several thousand patient care events reported to a malpractice insurance carrier. These events included poor outcomes without evident error, clear-cut errors, and patient complaints without evident error or injury. The fifth revision of the original taxonomy (version 01–0927) was further refined through the coding of approximately 350 ambulatory primary care medical errors (Fernald et al. 2004; Pace et al. 2005). Both the original taxonomy (Victoroff 2001) and the ASIPS modified version (http://fammed.uchsc.edu/carenet/asips/taxonomy) are available for review (www.errorsinmedicine.net). Recent improvements include the addition of a new axis to code error mitigation and recovery.

The DMO taxonomy includes 5 domains and 38 axes. Individual codes are arranged hierarchically within the 38 axes, ranging from 3-digit upper-level codes through 7-digit detailed, subordinate end codes. A fully coded event includes codes for all process steps (including causation), associated diagnoses, associated tests, associated medications, all participants, the outcome(s), the person(s) who discovered the event, and the setting(s). Mitigation and recovery codes are used only if these activities took place. Each event may be assigned several codes within each axis. Therefore, events can have a variable number of codes assigned. Users typically determine a minimum number of domains and axes to be used for a given project. For instance, the ambulatory project described above required a minimum of 10 codes to describe an event but averaged over 14 codes per event with a range of 10 to 44 codes for a single event.

The process orientation of the taxonomy is most evident in the domain 'Course of Event'. This domain is arranged according to the process problems, e.g., delay in performing a procedure, a procedure not performed, a procedure performed incorrectly. Detail of the clinical activity, e.g., lab process, imaging process, history taking, physical examination, is then coded at a deeper level of the taxonomy.

Through parallel construction the DMO taxonomy allows errors to be coded by process and clinical activity at the finest gradation while permitting facile grouping by process across various types of clinical activities or by clinical activity across various types of processes.

The International Taxonomy of Medical Errors in Primary Care (ITME-PC)

The AAFP/Linnaeus International Taxonomy of Medical Errors in Primary Care (ITME-PC) started as a data-driven taxonomy that has continued to evolve with further testing and influence by taxonomy theory. In 1999 the American Academy of Family Physicians investigated whether medical errors observed by family physicians in the United States could be adequately described by existing error taxonomies. The goal was to understand errors or mistakes ('anything that you see in your daily practice of medicine that should not happen') – not harms or adverse events. From a data set of 344 error reports submitted by family physicians in a 6-month period, it became apparent that a new structure for describing these errors was necessary. The AAFP taxonomy of medical errors grew from these data reports, using standard qualitative research techniques to develop descriptions of the types of errors reported and establish hierarchies of these descriptions (Dovey et al. 2002).

In 2001 this work was extended internationally through the Linnaeus Collaboration, a group of primary care researchers. General practitioners and family physicians in Australia, Canada, England, Germany, the Netherlands, New Zealand, and the United States reported 605 errors that were coded using the AAFP's taxonomy, which was freely modified and extended to accommodate the variety of reports coming from the seven different countries. Researchers in all seven countries were involved in the taxonomy development process that produced the AAFP/Linnaeus Taxonomy. This is a fairly complex taxonomy with a 6-level hierarchy in four domains encompassing error descriptions, contributory factors, consequences (including physical and emotional harm and harm severity, financial, time, and resource consequences) and prevention strategies. It is displayed in full in a paper file about 25 pages long.

Studies using the AAFP-Linnaeus taxonomy also collected data about errors that did not affect patients but instead involved healthcare providers (for example, needle stick injuries) or the care environment (for example, clinic cleanliness or lighting, refrigeration of vaccines). If a patient were involved in the event, the reporting system collected information about the doctor's familiarity with the patient, their age, sex, and whether they had a chronic or complex health condition. The taxonomy itself does not include these factors. Throughout its development, the ITME-PC has been tested using reports from primary care settings of error events observed there. Doctors, nurses, administrators, and students have all contributed reports.

Essential features of patient safety taxonomies

Despite their differences, each of these six taxonomies attempts to summarize the limited number of important features of patient safety events. Table 7.3 lists the primary domains or 'axes' of several patient safety taxonomies. Although different words are used to describe the domains, the concepts are very similar. Concepts not included in the first level of a taxonomy usually appear in the second level of the other taxonomies. We are in the early stages of patient safety taxonomy development, so there are likely to be many changes in all of these taxonomies, and efforts to collaborate and standardize are underway. Taxonomies will be evolutionary, not static, because of the constantly changing nature of medicine and technology, but the basic framework for the important issues affecting patient safety will stay reasonably stable regardless of location, healthcare setting, or specialty. Runciman's General Occurrence Model (Figure 7.1) for patient safety events provides an excellent model for developing any patient safety taxonomy, whether it be one designed to capture 'anything that goes wrong' in health care or for local or discipline-specific purposes (Aspden et al. 2004).

Table 7.3 The major domains (axes) of several patient safety taxonomies

NPSA	JCAHO PSET	ITME-PC	DMO
incident type	impact	error type	the patient
contributing factors	type	contributing factors	the outcome
severity of harm	domain	severity of harm	the course of the
service area	cause	actions taken	event
location	prevention and	consequences	the participants
staff type	mitigation	mitigating and	the observation
specialty		recovery factors	local codes (to be
medications		prevention	specified by the
devices		context variables (not	group using
		coded), including	the taxonomy)
		location, patient	
		demographics	

These are the essential issues one must consider in developing a patient safety taxonomy:

- Use a general theory-driven safety framework to organize the data. This differs from the approach of other scientific disciplines and many existing taxonomies that start with observations rather than theory.

- Use a relational database to allow for analyses of associations. This recommendation reflects the technology available to analyse data already organized according to a taxonomy.

- When feasible, use confidential reporting to allow detailed follow-up. This recommendation reflects the difficulty in obtaining full descriptions of 'events'.

- Examine mitigating and recovery factors.

- Incorporate a risk severity index to help direct improvement efforts.

- Consider the granularity issue: how many categories are enough to understand events?; too many categories impedes analyses. This is an issue for taxonomies across disciplines – as meaningful for the period table as for the most complex patient safety taxonomy.

- Develop a taxonomy that will allow the data to be rolled up into a general scheme for comparison with others. This refers to the value of using a single taxonomy to make comparisons across service areas, healthcare sites, organizations, and even countries. It is an issue specifically tackled in the work of the NPSA, JCAHO, and the Linnaeus Collaboration (above).

- Include events where no adverse outcomes occurred, as these help identify mitigating issues or agents in pathways that in other instances cause harm. This recommendation reflects the learning of the Runciman group but may not meet the goals of some other groups.

By following these principles, one is likely to devise a patient safety taxonomy that will provide maximum benefit in improving the safety of health care in any setting.

Future challenges

The patient safety taxonomies that we have presented here and others will compete in the political and economic marketplace. In some countries with national healthcare systems, it is likely that leaders will make decisions regarding the patient safety taxonomy to be used by their country. In countries like the United States that lack centralized healthcare systems and authority, many different patient safety taxonomies will continue to be used for local, regional and state regulatory and quality improvement goals. However, in the United States there is an active movement commissioned by the US Federal Government to the National Quality Forum (NQF) to identify and recommend a US national standard, and the JCAHO PSET taxonomy is the leading candidate.

Concurrent with these efforts is collaboration between JCAHO and the World Health Organization (WHO) to foster the International Safety Event Taxonomy

(IPSET) based on the PSET. In October 2004 the World Health Organization announced its plan to develop an international patient safety taxonomy that will

> serve to provide a uniform approach for linking the panoply of patient safety reporting activities undertaken in WHO Member States and to build a common information infrastructure for WHO to support initiatives to reduce medical errors and improve delivery of high-quality, safety care. The standards are being developed in order to ensure that those data most important to detecting, analyzing, understanding and learning from patient safety related events are comparable across existing reporting systems.
>
> (World Health Organization 2004)

Simultaneously, an international group of primary care researchers are independently working to develop a primary care taxonomy for patient safety that can be mapped to a general patient safety taxonomy such as the IPSET. This group has organized as a subcommittee of the World Organization of National Colleges and Academies of General Practice (WONCA) classification committee and will maintain a dialogue with the World Health Organization.

Box 7.1 Key points

- Classification systems exist to organize and display empirical findings in ways that aid or enhance our understanding. They are theoretical frameworks, not just ways to categorize or group data.
- Careful thought about the purpose of a patient safety taxonomy or classification system, guided both by theory and by practical experience, is needed. There is an interplay between the data and the concepts in design.
- Many adverse event reporting systems and patient safety taxonomies have sprung up, and most are homegrown classifications used in a limited number of organizations or systems. They tend to be empirically driven, by the data, and to have limited theoretical or conceptual grounding.
- Taxonomies will continue to evolve and develop, and it seems likely that a small number of widely accepted leading patient safety taxonomies will emerge, which will help to make data more comparable and lessons more transferable.
- The circumstances in which a taxonomy is used – for example, methods of reporting, the confidentiality of the process, and the response to reports – are just as important as the design of the taxonomy in determining its effectiveness.

References

Aspden, P., Corrigan, J.M., Wolcott, J. and Erickson, S.M. (eds) (2004) *Patient Safety: Achieving a New Standard for Care*. Washington, DC: National Academy Press, p. 297.

The ASIPS Collaborative: Dimensions of medical outcome. The ASIPS-Victoroff taxonomy. [Web page]. 2003; Available at http://fammed.uchsc.edu/carenet/asips/taxonomy/ (accessed July 16 2004).

Chang, A., Schyve, P.M., Croteau, R.J., O'Leary, D.S. and Loeb, J.M. (2005) The JCAHO patient safety event taxonomy: a standardized terminology and classification schema for near misses and adverse events, *International Journal for Quality in Health Care*, 17: 95–105.

Dovey, S.M., Meyers, D.S., Phillips, R.L., Green, L.A., Fryer, G.E., Galliher, J.M., Kappus, J. and Grob, P. (2002) A preliminary taxonomy of medical errors in family practice, *Quality and Safety in Health Care*, 11: 233–8.

Fernald, D.H., Pace, W.D., Harris, D.M., West, D.R., Main, D.S. and Westfall, J. (2004) Event reporting to a primary care patient safety reporting system: A report from the ASIPS Collaborative, *Annals of Family Medicine*, 2: 327–32.

Institute of Medicine Kohn, L.T., Corrigan, J.M. and Donaldson, M.S. (eds) (1999) *To Err is Human: Building a Safer Health System*. Washington, DC: National Academy Press.

Kaplan, H.S., Battles, J.B., Van der Schaaf, T.W., Shea, C.E. and Mercer, S.Q. (1998) Identification and classification of the causes of events in transfusion medicine, *Transfusion*, 38: 1071–81.

Norman, D.A. (1998) *The Psychology of Everyday Things*. New York: Basic Books.

Pace, W.D., Fernald, D.H., Harris, D., Dickinson, L.M., Main, D.S., Araya-Guerra, R. et al. (2005) Developing and analyzing a taxonomy to code ambulatory medical errors: a report from the ASIPS Collaborative. In *Advances in Patient Safety: From Research to Implementation*. Vol. 2. Concepts and Methodology. Henriksen, K., Battles, J.B., Marks, E.S. and Lewin, D.I. (eds). AHRQ Publication No. 05-0021-2. Rockville, MD: Agency for Healthcare Research and Quality; Feb. 2005.

Rasmussen, J. (1987) The definition of human error and a taxonomy for technical systems design, in *New Technology and Human Error*. London: John Wiley and Sons Ltd, pp. 23–30.

Reason, J. (1990) *Human Error*. Cambridge: Cambridge University Press.

Runciman, W.B. (2002) Lessons from the Australian patient safety foundation: setting up a national patient safety surveillance system – is this the right model?, *Quality and Safety in Health Care*, 11: 246–51.

Runciman, W.B., Helps, S.C., Sexton, E.J. and Malpass, A. (1998) A classification for incidents and accidents in the health-care system, *Journal of Quality Clinical Practice*, 18: 199–211.

Van der Schaaf, T.W.. Moraal, J. and Hale, A.R. (1992) Near miss reporting in the chemical process industry. Eindhoven, Netherlands: Technische Universiteit Eindhoven, Proefschrift.

Victoroff, M.S. (2001) Dimensions of medical outcome: a taxonomy. Version 01–0927 ('Five Decimal Version') Jointly developed and copyrighted with COPIC Insurance Company. [Web Page]. (Accessed 2005 September 15) Available at http://www.errorsinmedicine.net/taxonomy/asips/ASIPS_TAXONOMY_01_0927.pdf.

Victoroff, M.S. and Pace, W.D. (2003) Dimensions of patient safety: a taxonomy. Version ASIPS 650633600 – full. [Web Page] (Accessed 2005 September 15) Available at http://www.errorsinmedicine.net/taxonomy/asips/ASIPS_Victoroff_Taxonomy_650633600_full.pdf.

World Health Organization (2004) *World Alliance for Patient Safety: Forward Programme 2005*. Geneva: WHO.

8

Incident reporting and analysis

Sally Giles, Martin Fletcher, Maureen Baker and Richard Thomson

Incident reporting systems are emerging as a major tool to help identify patient safety problems and provide data for organizational and system learning. Much of their design is based on reporting systems, which have been successfully used in other high-risk industries for decades. This chapter presents an overview of incident reporting as a method of identifying Patient Safety Incidents (PSIs)[1] in health care. We explore the purpose of incident reporting and its growing importance. We review barriers to reporting and conclude with some challenges for the future. It is clear that incident reporting will, and indeed should, remain an integral part of the patient safety research and quality improvement agenda.

What is the purpose of incident reporting?

Incident reporting systems are primarily intended to help make health care safer for patients. Incident reporting typically involves healthcare staff actively recording information on events which have led to unintended harm or potential harm to patients. Incident reporting can also be used to document occurrences that are inconsistent with routine hospital operation, policies or procedures or evidence-based patient care (Dunn 2003). The process of incident reporting itself cannot improve the safety of patient care; rather, it is the response to the reports that is critical (World Health Organization 2004).

Reporting systems are based on the fact that most incidents involve a complex interplay of individual, team, technical and organizational factors (Barach and Small 2000). Although each incident is unique, there are likely to be similarities and patterns which may otherwise go unnoticed if incidents are not reported and analysed (Department of Health 2000). This might include factors such as communication problems, education and training, equipment and resources and team and social factors (National Patient Safety Agency 2004a). Awareness of the causes of, and contributing factors to such incidents is vital in order to identify gaps, inadequacies and weaknesses in the healthcare context in which incidents occur (Vincent 2004). Such insights can help to prevent major accidents, identify hazards within existing systems of care provision, identify new or rare events and generally help to understand the safety issues facing an organization or healthcare system (Barach and Small 2000; Department of Health 2000). One of the major aims of incident reporting is to gather qualitative data which can be used to promote learning alongside epidemiological data. This assumes that healthcare organizations can learn from others' experiences of adverse events and accidents (Department of Health 2000). This learning may be relevant at a number of levels including individuals and teams and general lessons which might be shared across organizations, regions and even whole countries (Department of Health 2000; Agency for Healthcare Research and Quality 2003; World Health Organization 2004). Box 8.1 describes an example of a PSI reported to an incident reporting system in primary care where the problem of misidentification of a patient is apparent. It highlights the potential for learning from incident reports at the interface of care. Although the patient came to no harm in this case, it shows that if healthcare professionals respond quickly to a PSI, they are more likely to be able to identify the potential for harm. Cases such as this one can provide an important mechanism for learning from PSIs and can reduce the risk of future re-occurrence.

To date, most incident reporting systems have been established at a local organizational level, particularly in acute care settings. Typically, data collected by local, organizational reporting systems are used to identify incidents which may require further investigation and to monitor organizational trends. Organizations may also use incident reports and investigations to inform organizational and system changes.

Increased interest in incident reporting

Incident reporting is by no means a new phenomenon. It has been used as an error prevention tool in many high-risk industries for decades. This includes aviation, nuclear power, petrochemical processing, steel production and military operations (Wald and Shojana 2001). More recently, it has gained in impetus within health care as a result of the findings of various studies investigating error rates, which have found that unintended patient harm is associated with around 3–17 per cent of hospital admissions (Brennan et al. 1991: Wilson et al. 1995: Gawande et al. 1999: Vincent et al. 1999). The potential human and financial cost of medical error has also increased interest in incident reporting. Indeed, it is estimated that medical error costs the US Government in the range of $29 billion annually and that there are up to 98,000 preventable deaths a year as a result of medical error (Institute of Medicine 1999). In the UK, it has been estimated that PSIs cost approximately £2 billion a year in additional hospital stays alone (Department of Health 2000).

As a result, establishing and improving incident reporting systems is a priority for many countries who want to develop national patient safety programs (Barach and Small 2000; World Health Organization 2004). There is increasing interest in the development of systems which receive reports from institutions and aggregate data at a regional, state or national level.

Incident reporting systems can come in many forms. This includes systems which focus on specific types of events (for example, blood transfusion events or sentinel events which lead to serious patient harm or death), areas of practice (for example, intensive care units) or across whole healthcare organizations (Wald and

---

Box 8.1 Incident reporting in primary care – a scenario (based on real experiences in primary care)

Mrs Jones is a 78-year-old who has been admitted to hospital following a myocardial infarction. She made a good recovery in hospital and has now been discharged home under the care of her GP, Dr Hindocha. At the end of morning surgery, Dr Hindocha receives a call from Nurse Davies, the district nurse attached to the practice. She has called in to assess Mrs Jones following her discharge from hospital. Nurse Davies has some queries regarding Mrs Jones's medication. Mrs Jones has no history of epilepsy, yet she appears to have been prescribed an anti-convulsant drug. She is also taking warfarin, an anti-coagulant, yet Mrs Jones does not appear to have any knowledge about why she is taking this medication or that regular monitoring, with blood tests, should be taking place. Dr Hindocha is equally puzzled. She retrieves Mrs Jones's discharge note and finds no mention of the anti-convulsant or anti-coagulation medicine having been prescribed. Dr Hindocha calls Nurse Davies and arranges to meet her at Mrs Jones's home so they can try to get to the bottom of what has happened.

By the time Dr Hindocha arrives at Mrs Jones's house, Nurse Davies feels she may have solved the mystery. The medication Mrs Jones took home from hospital is in the name of Dorothy Jones, but her first name is Doris. It would appear that their Mrs Jones – Doris – has been given another patient's medication on discharge. As her eyesight is poor, she did not notice that the medication was for Dorothy Jones. Moreover, she had been started on new drugs while in hospital and therefore was not familiar with her medication. Dr Hindocha and Nurse Davies are horrified at this mistake. They realize that either their patient, or the other lady involved, could have been harmed by taking the wrong medication. They would like to ensure that this situation does not happen again. However, they are not sure what steps they can take to do so.

Fortunately, their Primary Care Organization (PCO) has recently established an incident reporting system in an attempt to take a structured approach to learning from when things go wrong. If they submit a report about this incident, then the PCO can investigate the incident to try to determine what factors have led to this happening. It may be that the PCO has other reports of similar incidents, or other incidents occurring when patients have been discharged from this hospital. The information collected allows a structured approach to be taken in working with the hospital to improve procedures for discharge into the community. By reporting this incident locally, Nurse Davies and Dr Hindocha enable learning and action to occur, reducing the chance that such an event will happen again, to other patients.

Shojana 2001). Incident reporting systems may collect different sorts of data. For example, systems vary in the extent to which they capture information derived from any investigation of the root causes of an incident.

Incident reporting systems in health care have been subject to constant change. A recent focus of some local level incident reporting systems has been to establish electronic and web-based reporting. Box 8.2 describes an example of an electronic web-based incident reporting system in a three-star NHS Trust in Greater Manchester. This particular organization found that this type of system increased

---

Box 8.2 A case study of a local adverse incident reporting system (AIRS) in a 3-star NHS Trust in Greater Manchester

Brief description of the system and its development

This acute Trust introduced an electronic web-based incident reporting system in early 2002 with the option for the reporter to remain anonymous. The system allows anyone in the Trust to report a PSI from any available computer. It was designed in-house with the aim of simplifying the previous paper-based reporting system, reducing under-reporting and producing meaningful data that could be analysed statistically. It has recently been updated and it is now possible to report directly to the NRLS. The system currently receives, on average, 660 reports each month. There is no specific training for using the system. Members of staff in each division are shown how to use it at risk management training and expected to cascade the training down to other staff.

Process of reporting PSI to the system

Following a PSI, the incident form is completed on a webpage. The process of reporting and investigation is described below:

1. An incident form is completed on line.
2. The incident form is then placed on a list according to the specialty. Each specialty has a gatekeeper*, who can view a screen listing all PSI in their specialty. This list also indicates the severity of the PSI. The gatekeeper then nominates a suitable person to investigate the PSI.
3. The investigator receives an email asking them to investigate the PSI and a link to the investigation form.
4. Once the investigation is completed, the form is automatically sent to a clinical governance team to view. If they do not approve the report, it goes back to the investigator with comments and further work is then done, if required.
5. Once the report is accepted by the clinical governance team, it goes to risk management to be approved at a Trust level. If rejected, the original investigator is required to do more work on the report.
6. Once the report has been accepted by the risk management team, it becomes part of the incident reporting data.

*A person who is responsible for electing an appropriate person to investigate the PSI. They are not necessarily a senior person, but their work involves clinical governance.

---

their reporting levels by 60 per cent. They also found that this system had two major advantages over their previous paper-based system: first, it substantially reduced the time taken for incident reports to reach those investigating PSIs and, second, it allowed immediate access to the data for analysis. As with any incident reporting system, its success has primarily been driven by taking a low-blame approach, thus promoting more openness from health care staff.

Reporting systems may seek to address multiple objectives. This may include a focus on public accountability as well as learning. For example, ensuring that organizational action follows a serious patient safety incident. There is much debate about whether any one system can serve both learning and accountability purposes and about the tensions which may result from pursuing potentially contradictory objectives (Leape 2002), for example, use of incident data to assess the safety performance of an organization.

There is growing interest in reporting systems within primary care settings (Agency for Healthcare Research and Quality 2003; World Health Organization 2004). There is also an emerging focus on the role of patient reporting of incidents experienced during their own health care or that of a family member (National Patient Safety Agency 2004b). One of the major recommendations of the Kennedy Report into the Bristol Royal Infirmary was that patients should become more involved in the regulation of the safety and quality of their care (Department of Health 2001a).

Research evidence

In the past few years, reporting systems have been the subject of considerable research effort. However, in general, published studies have focused on whether incident reporting captures relevant events rather than seeking to establish the benefit of reporting in terms of patient outcomes or system changes (Agency for Healthcare Research and Quality 2003).

Research relating to incident reporting in both health care and other high-risk industries has identified some of the major factors associated with effectiveness. It has also highlighted some of the major problems and weaknesses. Of particular note, research suggests that under-reporting of patient safety incidents in health care is currently widespread (Barach and Small 2000; Wald and Shojana 2001). Table 8.1 summarizes some of the major barriers to incident reporting that have been identified through research.

Four inter-related themes emerge as important:

- *Open and fair culture.* Incident reporting occurs if the institutional environment is supportive and facilitates reporting. One of the major challenges is to establish

Table 8.1 Barriers to incident reporting

Fear of reprisal
Concerns about litigation
Concerns over anonymity
Ergonomics of incident reporting forms
Confusion over what constitutes an adverse event
Little immediate effect on improving quality of patient care
If nothing untoward happens as a result of an incident, there is no need to report
Lack of support from colleagues
Lack of feedback

Sources: Joshi et al. 2002; Wakefield et al. 1999; Vincent et al. 1999; Uribe et al. 2002; Kingston et al. 2004.

and maintain a positive safety culture within healthcare organizations. Health care is often associated with a weak safety culture (Singer et al. 2003). Sustained organizational leadership is an important element of creating a strong safety culture (National Patient Safety Agency 2004b). Other key elements include encouraging staff to report incidents, fairness in how incidents are dealt with, flexibility and a commitment to learning through a systems approach to analysing error rather than blaming individuals (Reason 1997; Department of Health 2000).

- *Safe to report.* Reporters may fear blame and punishment if they report incidents (Barach and Small 2000; National Patient Safety Agency 2004b). As a result, many reporting systems emphasize the importance of confidential or de-identified reporting (Department of Health 2001a). This typically involves a commitment not to identify the patient(s) or reporter to any third party. Reporting systems are often established at arm's length from regulatory bodies or those with powers to sanction the reporter or their organization (Leape 2002).

  There is continued debate about whether anonymity is an essential precondition to promote incident reporting (Runciman et al 2001; Kaplan and Barach 2002). A number of large-scale incident reporting systems are confidential and anonymous including the National Reporting and Learning System (NRLS) in England and Wales and the Australian Incident Monitoring System in Australia (AIMS). In some places and industries, confidentiality is accompanied by legislative or regulatory protection (Institute of Medicine 1999).

- *Coverage.* Most incident reporting systems recognize the importance of collecting information on a range of events. This includes major and minor injuries to patients, as well as near misses. Heinrich estimates a ratio in industry of one major injury and 29 minor injuries to 300 no-injury incidents (Department of Health 2000). Reporting systems in other industries have placed a particular emphasis on near miss reporting and analysis because similar patterns of error and system failures are often evident (Kaplan and Barach 2002). Similarly, in health care, near misses can provide important information about potential PSIs which can be used as a learning tool in order to prevent future occurrence. In practice, however, near miss reporting is not widespread (Giles et al. 2005).

  There is evidence of considerable confusion and debate among healthcare professionals over what constitutes a 'reportable' patient safety incident (Giles et al. 2004). Within individual healthcare organizations, there is often wide variation in definitions of reportable incidents (Dineen and Walshe 1999). Attitudes towards incident reporting are known to vary between professional groups (Kingston et al. 2004).

- *Worthwhile to report.* People will not report incidents if there is no perceived value in doing so. Various commentators have highlighted the importance of credible, expert and timely analysis of incident data involving people with 'operator expertise' of the work processes involved (Vincent 2004). Indeed, incident reporting has often been criticized for making inadequate use of any data produced and not focusing sufficiently on analysis in order to identify weakness which may pose threats to the safety of future patients (Vincent 2004). Research looking at incident reporting in the UK found that only 6 per cent of the participating hospitals were addressing the issue of using incident reporting data to improve quality of patient care (Dineen and Walshe 1999). Developments in analysis of incident data have also been accompanied by calls for common terminology and classification systems for determining risks (Runciman 2002; World Health Organization 2004).

Poor feedback is a major reason for under-reporting (Kingston et al. 2004). The need for rapid feedback to reporters and a means by which the reporting system can make recommendations and influence systems change are critical (Leape 2002; Runciman 2002). Ease of reporting is also important with increasing emphasis on electronic data collection systems (National Patient Safety Agency 2004a). Reporting systems in non-medical industries often provide incentives for voluntary reporting including rapid feedback to reporters (Barach and Small 2000).

Future challenges

Incident reporting systems within health care have been subject to steady change since their introduction. In part, this reflects the fact that approaches are being improved in the light of experience and the need for adaptation of approaches from other industries to suit the unique circumstances of health care.

We suggest three major challenges for the future. First is the need to try and reduce the extent of under-reporting of incidents by healthcare staff. This suggests a continued focus on strengthening the safety culture of healthcare organizations so that incident reporting has priority. This will require sustained attention to the range of barriers which have been identified. It will also require demonstrating the benefits of incident reporting. A key element of success will be to demonstrate how improvements in the safety of patient care have resulted from incident reporting and analysis. It will also be important to show that incident reporting is leading to action in relation to a range of contributing factors rather than a narrow focus on the behaviour and performance of the individual health care provider (Wald and Shojana 2001).

Second is an opportunity to explore the role of patients and their carers in reporting incidents. Patients may be able to provide information about their care that health care staff may not otherwise have known. For example, patients may experience an incident that may not be seen as such by the staff who work in the same environment from day to day. Indeed, it is known that if the same PSI occurs on a frequent basis, health care staff will stop reporting it, as it becomes 'normal' practice (Giles et al. 2005). As such, patient-initiated reports may have the potential to enrich the value of incident data for learning.

Third is the need to place incident reporting in a broader context. Done well, incident reporting will elicit information which provides a unique 'window' on the safety of patient care (Wald and Shojana 2001; Vincent 2004). However, incident reporting on its own will never provide a complete picture of all that may have gone wrong (Agency for Healthcare Research and Quality 2003). A multi-faceted approach to measurement, surveillance and risk management is needed. This may include activities such as data mining existing administrative and clinical data sets, regular reviews of medical records and staff and patient surveys which complement incident reporting (Agency for Healthcare Research and Quality 2003; National Patient Safety Agency 2004c).

This chapter has presented an overview of the current status and future challenges of incident reporting in health care. As healthcare systems strive to meet the challenge of improving patient safety and quality of care, it is clear that incident reporting has become an important tool and increasingly significant part of the healthcare policy agenda in many countries. Research suggests that in general there is a weak safety culture in healthcare organizations and, historically, health care staff have been reluctant to report patient safety incidents. A continued drive towards removing barriers to reporting is needed so that healthcare organizations can create an environment where healthcare staff feel both comfortable and safe when reporting incidents. Ultimately, success as a result of incident reporting will lie in being able to demonstrate that analysis stimulates learning and actions that lead to safer care for patients.

Note

1   Any unintended or unexpected incident which could have or did lead to harm for one or more patients receiving NHS-funded health care. This is also referred to as an adverse event/incident or clinical error, and includes near misses (Department of Health 2001c).

Box 8.3 Key points

- Data from incident reporting systems have huge potential to promote learning following PSIs and make care safer for future patients.
- In an attempt to improve quality of care and patient safety, incident reporting has become an increasingly significant part of healthcare policy agenda in many countries.
- Healthcare incident reporting systems are at an early stage of development and use compared to other high-risk industries.
- Effective incident reporting systems are reliant upon four major themes: (1) an open and fair culture; (2) an environment in which it is safe to report; (3) coverage of a range of incident types; and (4) making incident reporting worthwhile.
- A sustained drive towards removing barriers to reporting is needed so that healthcare organizations achieve an environment where healthcare staff feel both comfortable and safe reporting incidents.
- Ultimately, success as a result of incident reporting lies in being able to demonstrate continuous learning, analysis and action which leads to safer care for future patients.

References

Agency for Healthcare Research and Quality (2003) *AHRQ's Patient Safety Initiative: Building Foundations, Reducing Risk.* Interim Report to the Senate Committee on Appropriations. Rockville MD. http://www.ahrq.gov/qual/pscongrpt/ (accessed 17 Jan. 2005).

Australian Patient Safety Foundation www.apsf.net.au (accessed Dec. 2003).
Barach, P. and Small, S.D. (2000) Reporting and preventing medical mishaps: lessons from non-medical near miss reporting systems, *British Medical Journal*, 320: 759–63.
Brennan, T., Leape, L. et al. (1991) Incidence of adverse events and negligence in hospitalised patients: results of the Harvard Medical Practice Study I, *The New England Journal of Medicine*, February: 370–84.
Department of Health (2000) *An Organization with a Memory*. London: The Stationery Office.
Department of Health (2001a) *The Report of the Public Inquiry into Children's Heart Surgery at the Bristol Royal Infirmary 1984–1995*. London: The Stationery Office.
Department of Health (2001b) *Doing Less Harm: Improving the Safety and Quality of Care through Reporting, Analysing and Learning from Adverse Incidents involving NHS Patients. Key Requirements for Health Care Providers*. London: The Stationery Office.
Department of Health (2001c) *Building a Safer NHS for Patients*. London: The Stationery Office.
Dineen, M. and Walshe, K. (1999) Incident reporting in the NHS, *Health Care Risk Report*, 5(4): 20–2.
Dunn, D. (2003) Incident reports – their purpose and scope – Home study program, *AORN Journal*, July: 1–25.
Gawande, A.A., Thomas, E.J., Zinner, M.J. et al. (1999) Incidence and nature of surgical adverse events in Colorado and Utah in 1992, *Surgery*, 126(1): 66–75.
Giles, S.J., Cook, G.A., Jones, M.A. et al. (2004) Developing a list of adverse events for clinical incident reporting in Trauma and Orthopaedics, *Clinical Governance: An International Journal*, 9(4): 225–30.
Giles, S.J., Walshe, K., Cook, G.A. et al. (2005) Attitudes of health care professionals towards incident reporting (unpublished).
Institute of Medicine (1999) *To Err Is Human: Building a Safer Health System*. Washington, DC: National Academy Press.
Joshi, M.S., Anderson, J.F. et al. (2002) A systems approach to improving error reporting, *Journal of Healthcare Information Management*, 16(1): 40–5.
Kaplan, H. and Barach, P. (2002) Incident reporting: science or protoscience? Ten years later, *Quality and Safety in Health Care*, 11: 144–5.
Kingston, M.J., Evans, S.M., Smith, B.J. et al. (2004) Attitudes of doctors and nurses towards incident reporting: a qualitative analysis, *Medical Journal of Australia*, 181(5): 36–9.
Leape, L.L. (2002) Reporting of adverse events, *New England Journal of Medicine*, 347(20): 1633–8.
National Patient Safety Agency (2004a) *NRLS Service dataset -release version 1.2.1* www.npsa.nhs.uk/health/reporting/datasets (accessed 5 Feb. 2005).
National Patient Safety Agency (2004b) *Seven Steps to Patient Safety* www.npsa.nhs.uk/health/reporting/7steps (accessed 5 Feb. 2005).
National Patient Safety Agency (2004c) *Business Plan* www.npsa.nhs.uk/health/publications (accessed 5 Feb. 2005).
Nieva, V.F. and Sorra, J. (2003) Safety culture assessment: a tool for improving patient safety in healthcare organizations, *Quality and Safety in Health Care*, 12 (Suppl. 2): ii17–23.
Reason, J. (1997) *Managing the Risks of Organizational Accidents*. Aldershot: Ashgate.
Runciman, W. (2002) Lessons from the Australian Patient Safety Foundation: setting up a national patient safety surveillance system – is this the right model? *Quality and Safety in Healthcare*, 11: 246–51.
Runciman, W., Merry, A. and McCall Smith, A. (2001) Improving patients' safety by gathering information, *British Medical Journal*, 323: 298.

Singer, S.J., Gaba, D.M., Geppert, J.J. et al. (2003) The culture of safety: results of an organization-wide survey in 15 California hospitals, *Quality and Safety in Healthcare*, 12: 112–18.

Vincent, C. (2004) Analysis of clinical incidents: a window on the system not a search for root causes, *Quality and Safety in Health Care*, (13): 242–3.

Vincent, C., Stanhope, N. and Crowley-Murphy, M. (1999) Reasons for not reporting adverse incidents: an empirical study, *Journal for the Evaluation in Clinical Practice*, 5(1): 13–21.

Wakefield, D.S., Wakefield, B.J., Uden-Holman, T. et al. (1999) Understanding why medication administration errors may not be reported, *American Journal of Medical Quality*, 14(2): 81–8.

Wald, H. and Shojana, K.G. (2001) Incident reporting, in *Making Health Care Safer: A Critical Analysis of Patient Safety Practices*. Summary, July 2001. Rockville, MD: Agency for Healthcare Research and Quality, http://www.ahrq.gov/clinic/ptsafety/summary.htm (accessed 5 Feb. 2005).

Wilson, R., Runciman, W., Gibberd, R.W. et al. (1995) The Quality in Australian Health Care Study, *Medical Journal of Australia*, 164(12): 458–71.

World Health Organization (2004) *World Alliance for Patient Safety: Forward Programme 2005*. Geneva: WHO.

9
Using chart review and clinical databases to study medical error

Rachel L. Howard, Anthony J. Avery and Caroline J. Morris

Chart review and clinical databases have been used to study medical error in both primary and secondary care. The types of problems studied include preventable adverse events, and errors in the prescribing and monitoring of medication. Studies of preventable adverse events have contributed to policy on the safety of medical care. The US report, *To Err is Human: Building a Safer Health System* drew on the results of chart review studies conducted in New York, Utah and Colorado to illustrate the impact of preventable adverse events on patients admitted to hospital (Brennan et al. 1991; Leape et al. 1991; Institute of Medicine 1999; Thomas and Brennan 2000). In the United Kingdom, the Department of Health published *An Organization with a Memory*, which extrapolated from work carried out in the USA and Australia to illustrate the impact of adverse events on NHS patients (Brennan et al. 1991; Leape et al. 1991; Wilson et al. 1995; Department of Health 2000).

Chart review and clinical database studies have made a particular contribution to our understanding of medication-related problems. Medications are one of the most frequently used interventions in health care and all have the potential to cause injury (adverse drug events). These injuries can range from short-term illnesses such as nausea, to permanent disability or death. Some adverse drug events are due to the inappropriate use of medication and in some studies these are classified as 'errors'. In other studies the term 'preventable adverse drug event' is used instead. In order to understand the impact of preventable adverse drug events, it can be helpful to examine large populations in detail. This can be done using chart review or clinical database studies.

In this chapter we describe the contribution of large-scale chart review and clinical database studies to the medical error literature. We then describe the methods used in these studies and comment on their strengths and weaknesses. We illustrate these points using examples from large-scale studies that have been conducted throughout the world. Finally, we discuss the way forward for future studies using chart review and clinical databases.

The contribution of chart review and clinical database studies to the epidemiology of medical error

In primary care, studies have looked at preventable adverse drug events, and potential drug interactions in both ambulatory and nursing home patients. Methods used include chart review, interrogation of computer databases and patient surveys. Gandhi et al. (2003), using chart review and a patient survey, found that 3 per cent of patients in primary care experienced preventable adverse drug events following a new prescription. Gurwitz et al. (2003) combined chart review and computer alerts, and found 13.8 preventable adverse drug events per 1,000 person years. In another study in nursing homes, Gurwitz et al. (2000) found 0.96 preventable adverse drug events per 100 resident months.

Studies of drug interactions in primary care have been conducted in many countries using computer alerts. In the UK, Chen et al. (2005) found 4.3 per 1,000 patients on two or more medications were prescribed interacting drugs and a detailed review of 62 cases found that 44 cases were unjustified. In Finland, Sipila et al. (1995) found that 2.1 per cent of patients taking at least two drugs were using potentially harmful combinations, while in Sweden, Linnarsson (1993) found that 12 per cent of prescriptions for two or more drugs contained potential drug interactions.

In secondary care, retrospective chart review studies have been conducted in a number of countries, revealing differing rates of preventable adverse events. In the USA, the Harvard Medical Practice Study found that 3.7 per cent of hospital admissions were associated with adverse events; 58 per cent of these were associated with medical errors, but only 28 per cent of events were classified as negligent (Brennan et al. 1991; Leape et al. 1991). In a second US study from Utah and Colorado, Thomas and Brennan (2000) found that patients older than 65 years were twice as likely to suffer a preventable adverse event as younger patients (3.0 per cent vs 1.6 per cent). In the Quality in Australian Healthcare study, Wilson et al. (1995) found that 8.3 per cent of admissions were associated with high preventability adverse events, while in Canada, Baker et al. (2004) found only 2.8 per cent. In the UK, Vincent et al. (2001) found that 5.2 per cent of admissions were associated with preventable adverse events. Preventable drug-related admissions have also been studied throughout the world, and a systematic review of prospective chart review studies by Winterstein et al. (2002) has shown a median of 4.3 per cent of admissions to hospital are drug-related and preventable.

How chart review studies and clinical database studies are conducted

Chart review studies are manual reviews of medical records. They can include both electronic and paper prescription charts, and records from different care settings such as hospitals, accident and emergency departments and primary care records. Records are reviewed to extract relevant data, and then the records (or summaries of them) are assessed for causality and preventability. These assessments are often undertaken by more than one person to reduce the chance of misclassification. Large chart review studies are staff-intensive undertakings, and therefore expensive to conduct. The quality of data obtained from chart review studies depends on the quality of data recording, the people reviewing the information, and whether the data are viewed prospectively or retrospectively.

Clinical database studies are computer searches of electronic records for evidence of medical error. The quality of data obtained from clinical database studies depends on the accuracy and completeness of data recording and the design of appropriate search criteria (Morris et al. 2004). Search criteria can vary in complexity and trade-offs often have to be made between sensitivity and specificity.

Many studies have combined these two methodologies, using computer searches to identify medical records which may contain medical errors and then detailed manual review of the records to identify cases of medical error (Leape et al. 1995; Gurwitz et al. 2003; Chen et al. 2005).

Studies examining adverse events often define them as unintended injuries due to medical management (not the underlying disease) which result in measurable disability (Hiatt et al. 1989). The preventability of adverse events has been judged in a variety of ways, including whether there are signs of negligence, or if the injury could have been avoided by optimal medical care (Brennan et al. 1991; Howard et al. 2003). Adverse event studies measure only errors that have resulted in injury, while studies of errors in prescribing and monitoring medication can include patient injuries and 'near misses'.

Strengths and weaknesses of chart review studies

Below, we illustrate some of the strengths and weaknesses of chart review studies using examples of studies from the literature. One of these studies is the Harvard Medical Practice Study (HMPS) – the first large chart review study to assess adverse events in hospitals – sampling over 31,000 hospital records from 51 hospitals in New York state, using a methodology derived from the California Medical Insurance Feasibility Study (Hiatt et al. 1989). The methodology used in HMPS has subsequently been adapted, and we describe the effects of some of these changes on the reliability of these chart review studies in Box 9.1.

Quality of data

Medical records in secondary care are usually more detailed than those in primary care, often giving a daily summary of activities. In primary care, data recording is often brief, and intermittent, and is usually dependent on the patient consulting the physician. However, even in secondary care, data recording will be incomplete, and retrospective studies may under-estimate medical errors because of this. In the Quality in Australian Health Care study, Wilson et al. (1995) reported that only 73 per cent of medical records contained sufficient data to be able to identify adverse events and assess their preventability. Twenty-four suspected adverse events could not be assessed because there was insufficient data.

Retrospective versus prospective

Retrospective studies are, in many ways, easier to conduct, as the medical records can be reviewed away from the clinical area. In a retrospective study, however, there is no

---

Box 9.1 Changes to the HMPS methodology

The methodology developed in HMPS has been adapted and used in other large-scale chart review studies such as the Quality in Australian Healthcare Study (QAHCS), the Utah and Colorado Medical Practice Study (U&CMPS), a preliminary record review in UK hospitals, and the Canadian Adverse Events Study (CAES) (Wilson et al. 1995; Thomas et al. 2000; Vincent et al. 2001; Baker et al. 2004). In QAHCS, the following amendments were made to the methodology to improve reliability (Wilson et al. 1995):

- Nurse screeners of medical records underwent a 2-week intensive training course in the study protocols, and were provided with a review manual. A nurse team leader managed teams of screeners within each hospital.
- The nurse team leader reviewed a random selection of 50 records from each hospital to ensure that triggers were not being missed. There was 84 per cent nurse agreement on screening (kappa 0.67). This study also identified those criteria which showed the poorest agreement.
- The physician reviewers underwent a 2-day training course in the review technique and were provided with a review manual. Physician agreement on the presence of an adverse event was 80 per cent (kappa 0.55), but was only 58 per cent (kappa 0.33) for preventability.
- Where there was disagreement between two reviewers, they jointly re-reviewed the record, and presented their findings to a third reviewer.

The changes made in QAHCS appear to have improved the reliability of both the screening and the review process for preventability, compared to HMPS. However, it is important to note that agreement between reviewers is still low to moderate.

In U&CMPS, further amendments were made to the methodology, but despite efforts to improve the reliability of the review process, agreement between reviewers for the presence of an adverse event remained slightly worse than in HMPS and QAHCS (percentage agreement of 79 per cent; kappa 0.4 in U&CMPS vs 80 per cent; kappa 0.55 in QAHCS and 89 per cent; kappa 0.61 in HMPS) (Brennan et al. 1991; Wilson et al. 1995; Thomas et al. 2000).

---

opportunity to verify the information available, and records may be missing. Brennan et al. (1991) reported that the retrospective methodology used in HMPS meant that screeners were unable to access 4 per cent of the records identified for the study sample.

Prospective studies can allow for more comprehensive and detailed data capture by making efforts to clarify information from the medical records and to collect additional information. For example, this might include finding missing laboratory data or interviews with patients, relatives and staff members. In addition, many prospective chart review studies also include stimulated self-reporting of errors from healthcare staff, increasing the pick-up of errors.

Selection of screeners and reviewers

The quality of data obtained in a chart review study often depends on the person screening or reviewing the medical record. Data collected by untrained screeners and reviewers are often incomplete. Many studies have overcome this by training screeners and reviewers to ensure a consistent approach to case identification and assessment (Hiatt et al. 1989; Wilson et al. 1995; Thomas et al. 2000).

Screening records

Large chart review studies are a time-consuming and, therefore, costly process. Some studies rely solely on the case reviewers to screen all medical records to identify errors or adverse events. Other studies use healthcare professionals caring for the patients to identify potential adverse events (Howard et al. 2003; Pirmohamed et al. 2004). Other studies use trained screeners to identify medical records which meet specific criteria (a trigger tool) (Hiatt et al. 1989; Wilson et al. 1995; Thomas et al. 2000; Vincent et al. 2001; Baker et al. 2004). In studies where medical details are held electronically, the trigger tool can be a computerized search (Classen et al. 1997). In HMPS, nurses and medical-records administrators, trained to use a trigger tool, screened medical records for indicators of adverse events. The trigger tool included events such as previous hospitalization, drug reactions, death, indication of litigation and return to operating theatre (Hiatt et al. 1989). During the study, screeners failed to identify triggers in 11 per cent of records where they were present.

Assessment of records for presence of adverse events or errors

Once records have been highlighted, they can be reviewed in detail to identify adverse events or errors. This can involve reviewing the whole medical record, or a summary of the relevant data from the medical record (the latter avoiding problems with loss of medical records following screening). The review process usually involves an assessment of causality and preventability by trained medical, nursing or pharmacy personnel (depending on the types of events examined). The reliability of these assessments (and therefore of the study results) is judged by reviewer agreement.

Goldman (1992) has called into question peer review assessments of quality of care because the level of reviewer agreement is often little better than that expected by chance (assessed using the kappa statistic). Ashton et al. (1999) have shown that agreement is improved by the use of assessment criteria, either implicit guidance on the types of data to look for, or explicit guidance such as the algorithm developed by Naranjo et al. (1981) for assessing adverse drug reactions. Ashton et al. (1999) state that explicit guidance gives the best reviewer agreement.

Allowing reviewers to discuss their assessments does not improve the reliability of reviewer agreement. Hofer et al. (2000) showed that while agreement between reviewers was improved by discussion, the reliability of their assessments remained unchanged. Hayward and Hofer (2001) showed that low levels of agreement between reviewers also limited the reliability of assessments of preventability. In addition, Caplan et al. (1991) raised issues over the validity of physician review of preventability, finding that physicians were more likely to judge care as inappropriate if a case had a more severe outcome e.g. death vs disability.

In HMPS, medical records (rather than summaries of the records) were reviewed in detail. Attempts were made to improve the reliability of reviews by asking two physicians (from a possible 127) to perform detailed review of medical records containing possible adverse events, using implicit criteria to guide their assessments (Hiatt et al. 1989). Physician agreement was assessed by calculating percentage agreement and the kappa statistic (89 per cent agreement and kappa 0.61 for the presence of an adverse event; 93 per cent agreement and kappa 0.24 for the presence of negligence) indicating good agreement between physicians, but with a strong possibility that this agreement was a chance finding (Brennan et al. 1991). Localio et al. (1996) showed that physician agreement tended to be better where physicians had more experience in reviewing records, but this was not always the case. Also, physicians with high or low rates of adverse event identification tended to have the poorest agreement.

Chart review in drug-related admissions studies

Drug-related morbidity is considered to be a common cause of avoidable patient injury, with over 4 per cent of admissions judged to be preventable, and therefore associated with errors (Winterstein et al. 2002). Two large UK studies used prospective chart review methodologies to identify preventable drug-related admissions (Howard et al. 2003; Pirmohamed et al. 2004). Both studies used dedicated researchers, trained in chart review, to identify events. In addition, they asked healthcare practitioners to report suspected drug-related admissions (stimulated self-report) and gained more detailed data from patient and staff interviews. Both studies used structured implicit and explicit review to judge whether admissions had been caused by a drug-related problem (causality) and whether the admission could have been avoided (preventability). Those admissions judged as causal and preventable were considered to be due to medical error. Howard et al. (2003) reported greater reviewer agreement than that seen in studies of adverse events in secondary care (Wilson et al. 1995). Kappa statistics for pairs of reviewers ranged from 0.69 to 0.81 for assessments of causality and preventability, showing good agreement between reviewers. This may be a reflection of the narrower remit of the reviews, facilitating the use of structured review strategies.

Strengths and weaknesses of clinical database studies

Below, we describe some of the strengths and weaknesses of clinical database studies, using two studies to illustrate our points. In the first, Linnarsson (1993) identified potential drug interactions, which could be classified as prescribing errors. In the second, Honigman et al. (2001) compared four clinical database search methodologies, and their accuracy in identifying adverse events.

Resources required to undertake a clinical database study

Linnarsson (1993) suggested that clinical database studies are less time-consuming than chart review studies. This is because there is no need to employ and train chart screeners and reviewers, as the computer search performs both of these tasks. Therefore, these studies may be less expensive than research using chart review.

Quality of data in clinical databases

Not all healthcare agencies have electronic records. In the UK, electronic records are commonplace in primary care, but still unusual in secondary care. Those electronic records that are available have varying degrees of completeness. Many will not hold records of over-the-counter drugs, for example. As with retrospective chart review studies, this may lead to under-estimates in the rate of medical error. Linnarsson (1993) studied potential drug interactions in primary care using a clinical database search. He made no effort to verify whether actual harm had come to patients through these interactions.

Type of search employed

The type of search criteria employed in a database study is vital, as this will dictate the accuracy of data retrieval. This is clearly illustrated by Honigman et al. (2001) who compared the success of four search strategies of the Brigham Integrated Computer System, an electronic record of 88,514 ambulatory consultations by 15,564 patients, over one year. The search strategies were:

- Search for ICD-9 codes associated with adverse drug events (ICD-9 codes were entered at the end of each consultation).
- Search for medications prescribed to patients with a documented allergy to them.
- A trigger-tool methodology developed for the primary care setting, looking for new medication errors, abnormal laboratory results, and changes in laboratory results over time.
- Text searches linking drugs and drug classes to reported adverse effects.

The computer searches were then validated by detailed chart review of a sample of the highlighted records.
The positive predictive values (PPV) of the various search methods were:

- ICD-9 codes identified 214 incidents and had a low PPV of 0.02.
- Allergy rules identified 214 incidents, and had the highest PPV at 0.49.
- The trigger tool method identified 1,802 incidents, but had a low PPV of 0.03. Removing one rule with a low yield raised the PPV to 0.05, and three rules had a comparatively high yield for adverse events with PPVs ranging from 0.14 to 0.67.
- Text searching identified the most incidents (22,792) and adverse drug events, but also had a low PPV of 0.07.

Although this work was not specifically aimed at identifying errors, it does emphasize the need for carefully validated computer search terms and the additional need for chart review.

Specificity of the search employed

Studies of drug interactions rely on identifying two drugs being taken concurrently. Therefore, it is not enough to search a patient's record to see if two interacting drugs have been prescribed at any time. There must be a time limit set on the interval between prescribing the two drugs. Linnarsson (1993) set this time limit at one year, but also ensured that sufficient medication had been prescribed to cover that time interval. He also employed a more detailed search, to see if patients had been monitored appropriately while taking specific pairs of drugs. However, he was not able to elicit these data for all drug pairs.

Combining chart review and clinical database studies

Many investigators combine chart review and clinical database search methodologies to reduce the cost of identifying potential cases, while still enabling them to gain detailed information on individual cases. This methodology can be employed both prospectively and retrospectively. Gurwitz et al. (2003) combined computer-generated signals which identified toxic drug levels, clinical codes for poisonings, deranged blood tests and treatments for adverse drug effects with free-text searches of electronic records (as used by Honigman et al. (2001)) and manual chart review by clinical pharmacists to prospectively identify drug-related incidents occurring in primary care. Each search strategy identified different proportions of adverse drug events: 10.8 per cent from manual review of hospital discharge summaries; 12.1 per cent from manual review of emergency department notes; 28.7 per cent from computer signals and 37.1 per cent from automated free-text searching of the electronic record. Gurwitz et al. (2003) suggested that a periodic manual review of all medical records and interviews with patients (a method employed by Gandhi et al. (2003)) would have identified more adverse drug events.

Chen et al. (2005) used clinical database searches to retrospectively identify cases of potential drug interactions, and then performed a detailed chart review to identify whether harm had been caused to patients and whether the prescribed combination was intentional and appropriately monitored. Potential drug–drug and drug–disease interactions were identified in 90 patients. Detailed review of 62 medical records excluded 26 patients where the drugs had not been taken concurrently. In 21 patients the prescriber had documented that they were aware of the interaction at the time of prescribing, and in 14 cases the drug combination was thought to be appropriate.

Without access to detailed medical records, the investigators would have over-estimated the number of prescribing errors in the form of drug interactions. This need for detailed clinical information in the assessment of suspected medical error is further illustrated by the development of indicators of preventable drug-related morbidity (PDRM). PDRM is another term for preventable adverse drug events, and PDRM indicators have been used to identify specific types of injury caused by the inappropriate use of medication. Examples include administering painkillers with the potential to cause stomach bleeding (non-steroidal anti-inflammatory drugs) to patients who have had these problems in the past, or giving medications known to cause narrowing of the airways (bronchoconstriction) to patients with asthma, where this could result in serious morbidity or death.

Development of indicators of PDRM

Work conducted in both the North American and European healthcare systems has attempted to develop indicators that represent PDRM and to apply them in different patient databases. The original PDRM indicator set was developed in America using the Hepler and Strand (1990) definition of PDRM as its basis. For a drug-related morbidity to be preventable, the resulting adverse outcome or treatment failure must have been foreseeable and preceded by a recognizable drug-related problem that was both identifiable and controllable. Mackinnon and Hepler (2002) developed a series of indicators from an English-language literature review of peer-reviewed articles and referenced texts for types of preventable drug-related morbidity from 1967–98.

They were validated as representing PDRM using the Delphi consensus technique. Due to differences in clinical practice and prescribing patterns, direct translation of the American indicator set between countries cannot be automatically assumed. Researchers have therefore developed this work to produce indicator sets usable and relevant to their own healthcare contexts. To date, indicators have been developed for use in the Canadian, English and Portuguese healthcare systems.

In three of these systems, the indicators have been applied retrospectively in different primary and secondary care databases to help provide an indication of the extent of the problem and to identify the most commonly occurring PDRM events. In the future, it may also be possible to apply these indicators through databases or other information available in the community pharmacy setting.

Morris et al. (2004) have applied the indicators in electronic patient records in nine general practices in England. However, due to the complexity of the indicators, coupled with the technical difficulties in refining the computer searches to the degree required, a computerized approach alone is inadequate. To ensure valid and reliable data, an additional manual review of those records identified by computer searching is required.

Future challenges

Many of the studies included in this chapter have made a major contribution to the literature on medical error and their findings have been incorporated into policy documents to illustrate the size of the problem. There are, however, significant methodological issues with these studies. Simply using computerized searches of clinical databases will not elicit the required detail to make valid judgements about the causality and preventability of adverse events and medical errors. It is likely that future studies will continue to face methodological difficulties, and therefore it is important to be aware of the limitations of different approaches, and to try and ensure that future studies are designed to be as rigorous as possible.

Combinations of clinical database methodologies and chart review are likely to be the most sensitive techniques to identify medical errors in large studies and many possible search strategies are described in detail in the literature. However, the validity of identification methods should be carefully assessed in pilot work, prior to use in a large-scale study. Combining screening tools for use with clinical databases with prospective chart review will allow the collection of more detailed information from patients and healthcare professionals, while increasing the efficiency of data collection.

The reliability of studies of medical error is dependent on the levels of agreement between the reviewers assessing the presence of medical error. In the majority of studies, however, this agreement is poor to moderate. Much work has been done in this area, showing that agreement is better if explicit assessment criteria are used, and if reviewers receive the same training in using these criteria. Future studies need to take these factors into account.

Box 9.2 Key points

- Clinical database studies alone do not provide sufficient clinical information to judge the presence of medical error.
- Detailed clinical information is necessary to make judgements about the presence of medical error.
- Prospective studies allow collection of more complete datasets.
- Judgements on the presence of medical error vary greatly between reviewers. The use of explicit review criteria can reduce this variation, and hence increase study reliability.
- Providing the same training to all reviewers in the use of review criteria can increase reliability.
- Interviews with patients and healthcare professionals may increase the identification of medical error.
- Methodologies being transferred from other countries or healthcare settings should be adapted and validated in their new setting.

References

Ashton, C.M. et al. (1999) An empirical assessment of the validity of explicit and implicit process-of-care criteria for quality assessment, *Medical Care*, 37: 798–80.

Baker, G.R. et al. (2004) The Canadian Adverse Events Study: the incidence of adverse events among hospital patients in Canada, *Canadian Medical Association Journal*, 170: 1678–9.

Brennan, T.A. et al. (1991) Incidence of adverse events and negligence in hospitalized patients: Results of the Harvard Medical Practice Study I, *The New England Journal of Medicine*, 324: 370–6.

Caplan, R.A. et al. (1991) Effect of outcome on physician judgements of appropriateness of care, *Journal of the American Medical Association*, 265: 1957–60.

Chen, Y-F. et al. (2005) Incidence and possible causes of prescribing potentially hazardous/ contraindicated drug combinations in general practice, *Drug Safety*, 28: 67–80.

Classen, D.C. et al. (1997) Adverse drug events in hospitalized patients: excess length of stay, extra costs, and attributable mortality, *Journal of the American Medical Association*, 277: 301–6.

Department of Health (2000) *An Organization with a Memory*. London: Department of Health.

Gandhi, T.K. et al. (2003) Adverse drug events in ambulatory care, *New England Journal of Medicine*, 348: 1556–64.

Goldman, R.L. (1992) The reliability of peer assessments of quality of care, *Journal of the American Medical Association*, 267: 958–60.

Gurwitz, J.H. et al. (2000) Incidence and preventability of adverse drug events in nursing homes, *American Journal of Medicine*, 109: 87–94.

Gurwitz, J.H. et al. (2003) Incidence and preventability of adverse drug events among older persons in the ambulatory setting, *Journal of the American Medical Association*, 289: 1107–16.

Hayward, R.A. and Hofer, T.P. (2001) Estimating hospital deaths due to medical errors: preventability is in the eye of the reviewer, *Journal of the American Medical Association*, 286: 415–20.

Hepler, C.D. and Strand, L.M. (1990) Opportunities and responsibilities in pharmaceutical care, *American Journal of Hospital Pharmacy*, 47: 533–43.

Hiatt, H.H. et al. (1989) A study of medical injury and medical malpractice: an overview, *New England Journal of Medicine*, 321: 480–4.

Hofer, T.P. et al. (2000) Discussion between reviewers does not improve reliability of peer review of hospital quality, *Medical Care*, 38: 152–61.

Honigman, B. et al. (2001) Using computerized data to identify adverse drug events in outpatients, *Journal of the American Medical Informatics Association*, 8: 254–66.

Howard, R.L. et al. (2003) Investigation into the reasons for preventable drug related admissions to a medical admissions unit: observational study, *Quality and Safety in Health Care*, 12: 280–5.

Institute of Medicine (1999) *To Err is Human: Building a Safer Health System*. Washington DC: National Academy Press.

Leape, L.L. et al. (1991) The nature of adverse events in hospitalized patients: Results of the Harvard Medical Practice Study II, *The New England Journal of Medicine*, 324: 377–84.

Leape, L.L. et al. (1995) Systems analysis of adverse drug events, *Journal of the American Medical Association*, 274: 35–43.

Linnarsson, R. (1993) Drug interactions in primary health care, *Scandinavian Journal of Primary Health Care*, 11: 181–6.

Localio, A.R. et al. (1996) Identifying adverse events caused by medical care: degree of physician agreement in a retrospective chart review, *Annals of Internal Medicine*, 125: 457–64.

Mackinnon, N.J. and Hepler, C.D. (2002) Preventable drug-related morbidity in older adults: 1. Indicator development, *Journal of Managed Care Pharmacy*, 8: 365–71.

Morris, C.J. et al. (2004) Indicators for preventable drug related morbidity: application in primary care, *Quality and Safety in Health Care*, 13: 181–5.

Naranjo, C.A. et al. (1981) A method for estimating the probability of adverse drug reactions, *Clinical Pharmacology and Therapeutics*, 30: 239–45.

Pirmohamed, M. et al. (2004) Adverse drug reactions as cause of admission to hospital: prospective analysis of 18 820 patients, *British Medical Journal*, 329: 15–19.

Sipila, J. et al. (1995) Occurrence of potentially harmful drug combinations among Finnish primary care patients, *International Pharmacy Journal*, 9: 104–7.

Thomas, E.J. and Brennan, T.A. (2000) Incidence and types of preventable adverse events in elderly patients: population based review of medical records, *British Medical Journal*, 320: 741–4.

Thomas, E.J. et al. (2000) Incidence and types of adverse events and negligent care in Utah and Colorado, *Medical Care*, 38: 261–71.

Vincent, C. et al. (2001) Adverse events in British hospitals: preliminary retrospective record review, *British Medical Journal*, 322: 517–19.

Wilson McL, R. et al. (1995) The Quality in Australian Health Care Study, *Medical Journal of Australia*, 163: 458–71.

Winterstein, A.G. et al. (2002) Preventable drug-related hospital admissions, *Annals of Pharmacotherapy*, 36: 1238–48.

10
Techniques used in the investigation and analysis of critical incidents in health care

Stephen Rogers, Sally Taylor-Adams and Maria Woloshynowych

Important theoretical insights are fuelling developments in accident prevention in various fields. However, the literature on the investigation and analysis of critical incidents in health care remains diverse and poorly integrated. In particular, there has been little effort to map different approaches. In our view, six core techniques provide a useful foundation for making comparisons between approaches. In this chapter we provide a descriptive summary of each of these techniques. For each technique we describe the background essential features and theoretical basis. We also set out its application in health care and explore its strengths and limitations. Then we provide an assessment of the techniques against a predefined set of criteria for the evaluation of accident investigation methods (Benner 1985; Kirwan 1992) and discuss the implications for continuing development and application of accident investigation and analysis techniques in health care.

The six core techniques discussed here are:

1. Australian Incident Monitoring System (AIMS).
2. Confidential inquiry method (CIM).
3. Critical incident technique.
4. Significant event auditing (SEA).
5. Root Cause Analysis (RCA).
6. Organizational Accident Causation Model (OACM).

Australian Incident Monitoring System (AIMS)

The origin of AIMS derives from an incident monitoring study in anaesthesia (AIMS-Anaesthesia) that began in 1988. The system was subsequently expanded for use on an institutional basis and AIMS now provides a mechanism for any incident (actual or potential) to be reported, using a single standard form. AIMS is run by the Australian National Patient Safety Foundation (APSF), a non-profit-making independent organization for promoting patient safety. The system is currently implemented in several Australian States, and individual health units. In 2000 the system was piloted in New Zealand and has subsequently informed the development of the National Reporting and Learning System implemented by the National Patient Safety Agency in the United Kingdom.

Incident information is collected on a paper form and data are entered and coded using dedicated software. Data from AIMS are classified using the Generic Occurrence Classification (GOC), a classification that evolved directly from AIMS data. In essence, this is a large tree structure with multiple choices at a number of levels. The AIMS software elicits the key clinical information, places the event in context and records the contributing factors, both system-based errors and human errors. Some of the contributing factors that are recorded include: management decisions; infrastructure, working conditions; communications, records; staff quantity and quality; supervision and tasking; equipment availability and/or suitability; policies, protocols and pathways. The coding of the information provides the method of understanding the underlying causes of the incident and of analysing the contributory factors and supports the preparation of a range of comprehensive reports to assist management in identifying problems and remedial action.

Runciman's model allows for an error to occur anywhere in the chain from intention, through planning action to outcome and draws on Norman's slip/mistake distinction, Reason's categories of knowledge-based mistakes, rule-based mistakes and skill-based slips and lapses, along with the conceptual framework put forward by Rasmussen (Runciman et al. 1993).

The majority of published studies are in anaesthetics or intensive care, with additional studies carried out in family practice, psychiatry, intensive care and obstetrics (e.g. Sinclair et al. 1999; Steven et al. 1999; Morris and Morris 2000). All studies rely on individuals, usually clinicians or nursing staff, voluntarily reporting incidents and typically data are analysed by individuals working outside the organizations involved. Although a majority of publications are from Australia, researchers have also published results of studies using AIMS-type approaches in New Zealand (Kluger and Short 1999) and in a number of Asian countries (e.g. Chen et al. 1998; Choy et al. 1999).

AIMS provides a national and international system that enables comparative data analysis, identification of common factors and trends from aggregated data. Such identification can help in justifying changes or proposals that require funding. The system ensures anonymity so that staff are more likely to report incidents and in Australia there is some legal protection against disclosure in information in reports. However, the level of information is dependent on the amount of detail provided by the person reporting the incident. Only one type of data is collected and analysed (secondary documentation) giving no opportunity to check accuracy and it is usually not possible to further investigate a particular incident because of informant protection.

Confidential inquiry method (CIM)

The application of the audit approach to the problem of maternal deaths was instituted in the United Kingdom in 1952, preceding the institutionalization of audit as a quality improvement technique in other areas of health care. National confidential inquiries were initiated subsequently for the investigation of peri-operative deaths, the investigation of stillbirths and deaths in infancy and the investigation of suicide and homicide in people with mental illness. At the time of writing, the confidential inquiry model has been used to investigate healthcare quality in many countries and across a broad range of healthcare problems.

Confidential inquiries have basic similarities in the way they are conceptualized and conducted. Typically, efforts are made to identify all incidents of interest (usually deaths) in a defined population over a specified time period. Statutory systems for certification of deaths, voluntary notification (especially enquiries into perinatal mortality) and, in less developed countries, hospital and community-based enquiries provide the cases for study. Medical records are usually examined to ascertain the details of the case, and the approach may be supplemented by questionnaire enquiries or interviews with healthcare staff or relatives. Individuals, or groups who are experts in their field, assess the information assembled against implicit or explicit standards for care. Detailed publications are produced for national confidential enquiries, including tabulations of findings and recommendations for improvements. Typically, confidential enquiries focus on clinical and patho-physiological and some studies have included a meaningful focus on organizational issues (Drife 1999).

The underlying theoretical assumption for audit is that healthcare staff and healthcare managers want to perform well, but have little appreciation of the standard of their own performance. Audit with feedback is considered to be a behaviour modification approach where demonstration of underperformance or deficiencies in care is expected to drive change in the behaviour of individuals and groups (Balcazar et al. 1985).

The majority of publications are derived from confidential enquiries into maternal, perinatal or post-operative deaths (e.g. Wood et al. 1984; Walker et al. 1986; Cartlidge et al. 1999) but there are many examples of the same approach being applied to other problems such as deaths from strokes, hypertension or asthma (Payne et al. 1993; Burr et al. 1999) and to problems in less developed country settings (e.g. Walker et al. 1986; Durrheim et al. 1999).

The confidential approach and voluntary participation are reassuring for clinicians who might worry about professional credibility and litigation. Close involvement of professional organizations helps to endorse ownership by participants and to institutionalize involvement without the need for statute. Complete ascertainment of cases improves generalizability of findings and enables meaningful links to be made with denominator populations at risk of the adverse outcome. Use of standardized data collection methods enables comparable data collection across sites and over time, and analysis at regional as well as local level promotes local review and implementation of change. The main limitations of the approach are that confidential inquiries have tended to focus on clinical activity rather than on contextual issues, which might determine patient safety. Due to issues of scale, it is only feasible to conduct serial confidential enquiries for a relatively small number of adverse outcomes of significant public health importance. The findings of confidential enquiries are remote from individual cases and their influence on implementation of change is mainly through dissemination of findings via professional organizations and scientific literature.

Critical incident technique

The critical incident technique (CIT) was first described by Flanagan (1954) who set out a series of defined steps for collecting and analysing critical incidents. The true ancestor of most healthcare papers is Cooper's (Cooper et al. 1978) study on preventable anaesthetic mishaps, using a modification of the critical incident technique. With some exceptions (Waterston 1988; Bradley 1992), the methods of most healthcare studies are closer to those of Cooper than to Flanagan and we use Cooper's paper as our model for the critical incident technique in health care.

Clinicians of the relevant specialty have carried out most studies, relying primarily on interviews following voluntary incident reporting. Early studies (Cooper et al. 1978, 1984) used interviews with members of staff and in a second phase moved on to paper-based methods. The nature of the interviews has not usually been well specified, and where questionnaires have been used, few details were given. Cooper et al. (1984) describes the search for causal patterns as 'primarily an intuitive process'. Incidents were broadly classified as human or equipment error, types of human error, by the nature of the activity, the nature of the problem occurring (e.g. disconnection, drug overdose), severity of outcome. Cooper also discusses 'associated factors', such as fatigue or inadequate experience, which describe circumstances that may have contributed to the error or adverse outcome and provides a table of strategies for prevention of incidents based not only on the specific clinical problems identified but also on the more general problems underlying a number of different kinds of errors. Cooper, reflecting on the impact of these studies, noted that 'they seem to have stirred the anaesthesia community into recognizing the frequency of human error in the specialty and generated great interest in reducing the rate of mistakes by instituting many different preventative strategies'.

No specific theoretical basis is adduced for critical incident studies, although the work of Flanagan is routinely acknowledged. Cooper's work substantially extends the traditional approach, drawing as it does on human factors work and the psychology of human error.

The original anaesthetic critical incident studies have been duplicated in the UK, the Netherlands and Australia and were influential in the formation of the AIMS project. Outside anaesthesia studies have been carried out in intensive care (Wright et al. 1991), on deaths in general practice (Berlin et al. 1992), and uncomfortable prescribing decisions (Bradley 1992).

The critical incident technique as described by Flanagan provides a research-based approach for the investigation and analysis of clinical incidents. Used as specified, the approach allows information on causes and contributory factors to emerge as cases are gathered, and has validity as a qualitative research method utilizing grounded analysis. Modifications of the approach, using smaller numbers of interviews, paper-based accounts and classifications that are partly predetermined are more pragmatic, but risk accuracy in the way that classifications are formulated. Only anaesthetics has produced a sustained series of studies in which an understanding of the causes of incidents has been followed by the introduction of preventative measures.

Significant event auditing (SEA)

Significant event auditing (SEA) involves reflection on the circumstances of a single case or event, with adverse, or sometimes with successful outcomes (Pringle et al. 1995). SEA has been defined as a process in which individual episodes are analysed in a systematic and detailed way to indicate what can be learned about the overall quality of care and to indicate changes that might lead to future improvements (Pringle et al. 1995). It is widely used as an educational approach in the general practice setting in the United Kingdom, where adverse events including deaths, patient complaints or administrative mistakes may be used as a starting point for significant event auditing.

In practice, SEA meetings are conducted in groups as a work-based reflective activity. The effective functioning of the group is generally accepted as a prerequisite for successful significant event auditing (Robinson et al. 1995). One member of the team presents the details of an incident and leads the SEA process (Westcott et al. 2000) or an outsider, skilled in managing small groupwork, facilitates the process (Robinson et al. 1995). Pringle et al. (1995) suggest that any significant event meeting should include consideration of: the immediate management of the case; the possibilities for prevention; the implications for family or community; interface issues; team issues; action to be taken or policy decisions to be made; and follow-up arrangements. With a few exceptions (Pringle et al. 1995), written reports generated by SEA are retained, rather than disseminated for wider learning.

There is no explicit link to theories of accident causation. Significant event auditing is often said to be derived from the critical incident method developed by Flanagan (1954) but, in our view, these methodological links are tenuous. For example, individual interviews are used in Flanagan's work with cumulative classification of data collected across multiple cases, while SEA is group-based, standards are judged by peer review and learning is usually from single or a small series of cases.

SEA is actively promoted as a vehicle for quality improvement in the UK general practice setting (Pringle et al. 1995). Most publications describe development or evaluation of the method, with a few including information on actual cases studied (e.g. Westcott 2000). The approach has nevertheless been extended to explore quality problems in palliative care (Bennett and Danczak 1994) and mental health care (Redpath et al. 1997).

Many potential benefits such as the ability to stimulate clinical audit, to inform commissioning and improve quality have been documented (Pringle et al. 1995; Pringle 1998). SEA can improve the morale of primary care teams, improve communication and working environments, but only if it is sensitively and effectively managed (Westcott et al. 2000). However, the process does need to be actively managed if it is to be successful. In Westcott's (2000) study, there were difficulties finding time and ensuring ongoing support for meetings, concerns about boundaries and, for some staff, concern about speaking out, particularly when all the topics came from one professional group, such as the doctors. Problem analysis in SEA is sometimes superficial. The process may identify issues at the level of individuals or practice systems and the generation of action points is intrinsic to the SEA, but the degree to which SEA activities have actually led to implementation of change in practice has not been systematically evaluated.

Root Cause Analysis (RCA)

Root Cause Analysis (RCA) was developed more than 30 years ago as a methodology to investigate serious accidents in the industrial sector. In the health sector, the Joint Commission on Accreditation of Healthcare Organizations (JCAHO) in the USA developed an RCA model to investigate 20 sentinel events in health care and there is now an international interest in using this approach, fuelled by the publication of key documents such as *Organization with a Memory* (Department of Health 2000), and *Making Healthcare Safer* (2001) in the UK. The National Patient Safety Agency (NPSA) has subsequently designed and developed a comprehensive approach to RCA and an associated training programme for all healthcare providers in England and Wales.

The JCAHO (2000) document provided the first comprehensive guide on how to complete a successful RCA. It is based on 21 separate steps and provides examples of 14 RCA tools which makes it an extremely thorough approach. Others have taken a simplified approach, where many of the component steps have been integrated, e.g. Amo (1998) identified seven steps in RCA and Handley (2000) refined the process further, reducing it to just five. The NPSA's model of RCA focuses on 10 stages comprising:

1 Report incident.

2 Decision to investigate and setting up investigation team.

3 Gather data.

4 Map chronology.

5 Identify care/service delivery problems.

6 Identify contributory factors and root causes.

7 Develop recommendations.

8 Write report.

9 Implement solutions.

10 Evaluate and audit solutions.

The NPSA model provides information on 13 associated tools. JCAHO and the NPSA also provide a number of useful worksheets, templates and tables for undertaking an RCA and the NPSA has developed an e-learning toolkit for RCA as a free resource to the service.

RCA is essentially a total quality management tool. It is a systematic approach that drills down deep to identify the basic reason(s) for a problem – the root cause(s). The analysis repeatedly digs deeper by asking 'why?' questions until no additional logical answer can be found and identifies changes that could be made in systems or processes that would improve performance and reduce the risk of a particular serious adverse event occurring in the future. Classic RCA is not based on any specific theory of human error or system failure though the NPSA's RCA makes some explicit links to Reason's organizational accident causation model and Rasmussen's skills, rule and knowledge model.

RCA has been applied to a variety of medical specialties and problems, e.g. drug overdose during cancer therapy, blood transfusion reactions in ICU, laboratory delays to an A&E department, independent mental health homicide inquiries. Many papers (e.g. Beyea and Nicoll 1999; Berry and Krizek 2000; Shinn 2000) focus on the early stages of the RCA process, e.g. setting up a team and collecting the factual information to support a full investigation. These papers only seem to discuss a few RCA tools e.g. brainstorming and the cause and effect chart, Pareto charts and time-lines. Hirsch and Wallace (1999) outline the use of contributory factor trees (also known as fishbone diagrams), and taxonomies to identify contributory factors and root cause(s) of an adverse event. RCA is currently being applied extensively at a local level within healthcare incidents.

RCA is directed towards identifying weak points in systems, and a focus on how to improve systems rather than blaming an individual. RCA provides investigators with a complete accident methodology, utilizing a variety of techniques to investigate and analyse error. Limited documentation exists in the healthcare sector on the range of RCA tools available and in particular worked examples showing their applicability to certain types of accident investigations. Accident investigators must be fully trained in a variety of RCA techniques if they are to successfully analyse incidents. RCA can very easily be made overly complicated and does not guarantee a complete answer. Also RCA can be a time-consuming process, if a variety of detailed techniques are used.

Organizational Accident Causation Model (OACM)

Studies that have based their investigation and analysis of critical incidents on Reason's Organizational Accident Causation Model (Reason 1997, 2001) include the approach of Vincent et al. (1999), Eagle et al. (1992) and the Winnipeg model (Davies 2000). Vincent (1999) and colleagues developed a generic protocol for the investigation and analysis of serious incidents in health care, which has since been tested in various settings. This model is now well accepted in the UK and the classification system of contributing factors proposed has been incorporated (but also extended) into the National Patient Safety Agency's (NPSA) RCA toolkit.

The protocol gives a detailed account of the investigation and analysis process (Vincent et al. 1999). Accounts of an incident may be taken from written reports of staff members, case notes or interviews with staff. The essential process of investigation and analysis is mirrored in the structure of the interviews. The aims of the interview are as follows: (1) to establish the chronology, including the role of the member of staff being interviewed and their account or experience of the events; (2) to identify the 'care delivery problem' (CDP) or actions or omissions made by staff or other limitations in the system that had an important role in the critical incident; and (3) to present a framework of contributory factors that is applied to each CDP identified, and is discussed with the interviewee to identify the most important factors and potential methods of prevention. The end result is a report that summarizes the chronology of the incident, identifies all CDPs and associated contributory factors, reports the positive features of the process of care and recommends action with time-scales for each general factor requiring attention.

The Organizational Accident Causation Model developed by Reason (1997, 2001) illustrates how fallible decisions at the higher echelons of the management structure or latent failures have an effect at departmental levels, where task and environmental conditions can promote unsafe acts. Defences and barriers are designed to protect against hazards and to mitigate the consequences of equipment and human failure. In an investigation, each of these elements is considered in further detail, starting with the failed defences and working backwards to the root organizational processes.

Appraisal of key papers in health care shows that studies have been conducted in a number of different settings including nursing, psychiatry, obstetrics, intensive care, anaesthetics and surgery (e.g., Stanhope et al. 1997; Vincent et al. 2000). The focus of such studies has tended to be on illustrative cases, although recent studies consider larger numbers of cases. Investigations have depended on interviews, with some confirmation of events or details from the medical records. The pattern was for the conduct of individual, semi-structured interviews with a number of staff from a range of disciplines. In some studies, a checklist of contributing factors was used (Stanhope et al. 1997).

OACM focuses on improving systems and the working environment rather than blaming individuals and is based on current accepted models of human performance. The approach identifies a range of weakness in systems, teams and/or individuals and publications are available that can provide investigators with a complete investigation tool. Nevertheless, the models and theories on which the methods are based have not been formally evaluated and investigators have had difficulty with some of the terminology. Although the techniques have been used in investigations, there is little documentation of findings being used to inform specific interventions.

Assessment of techniques against evaluation criteria

Each technique was assessed against a pre-defined set of criteria based on items specified by Benner (1985) and Kirwan (1992) for the evaluation of accident investigation methods. A full description of the exercise appears elsewhere (Woloshynowych et al. 2005) and a detailed description of the assessment criteria appears in Box 10.1.

Criteria cover the validity of methods based on theoretical foundations and whether human and organizational factors are incorporated and the likely consistency (and thus accuracy) of their application. Other criteria address whether the findings are likely to be comprehensive in their consideration of errors and independent in the sense that they produce blameless outputs. Consistency in the interpretation of the facts is considered and whether the investigative process is likely to be auditable. Then, the probable usefulness of the method is gauged and the likely acceptability of the approach overall is considered.

Model-based validity was high only for OACM and moderately so for AIMS. All methods tended to have limitations in the degree to which they illustrated the what, how and why questions relevant to the understanding of accidents. For example,

Box 10.1 Assessment criteria for critical incident techniques

Comprehensive – is defined by the following three criteria:

1 Accuracy of identifying significant errors (i.e. those which have the most impact on risk).
2 Breadth of coverage of the technique in dealing with all forms of error.
3 Ability to identify all possible errors given the task and task environment.

Low comprehensiveness (0) = fails to satisfy any comprehensive criteria or only one.
Moderate comprehensiveness (1) = satisfies at least two of the above criteria.
High comprehensiveness (2) = satisfies all three of the above criteria.

Consistent – degree to which different assessors utilize the methodology in the same way and thus is more likely to yield consistency of results, verses an open-ended methodology, in which the results are likely to be highly assessor-dependent.

Low consistency (0) = relatively open-ended method.
Moderate consistency (1) = assessor has flexibility within a detailed framework.
High consistency (2) = tool is highly structured and therefore likely to lead different assessors to same result.

Theoretical Validity (Model based) – whether approach is based on an accident model or theory of human behaviour/performance.

Low theoretical validity (0) = just a classification system.
Moderate theoretical validity (1) = technique makes reference to a model.
High theoretical validity (2) = tool is the embodiment of model.

Theoretical validity – whether the technique simply assesses External Error Modes (EEM) – what happened; whether it also identifies Psychological Error Mechanisms (PEM) – how it happened; and Performance Influencing Factors (PIF) – why it happened.

Low theoretical validity (0) = either does not consider EEM, PIF or PEM or only one of these components.
Moderate theoretical validity (1) = considers two of the above three components.
High theoretical validity (2) = considers EEM, PEM and PIF.

Error reduction (usefulness) – the degree to which the technique can generate error reduction mechanisms.

Low usefulness (0) = technique has little concern for error reduction.
Moderate usefulness (1) = technique is capable of error reduction.
High usefulness (2) = error reduction is a primary focus of approach.

Resources (usage) – likely resource usage in actually applying technique, in terms of assessor or experiment time. Resources were rated either as low, moderate or high depending on the judged extent of time each technique would take to apply.

Low resources (0) = technique takes less than one day to apply.
Moderate resources (1) = technique takes between one day and one week to apply.
High resources (2) = technique takes more than one week to apply.

Auditable documentation – the degree to which the technique lends itself to auditable documentation.

Low documentability (0) = utilization of technique is difficult to document.
Moderate documentability (1) = technique provides sufficient documentation to be repeatable.
High documentability (2) = all assumptions are recorded and documentation is useful for future system operations.

Independence – methodology must produce blameless outputs. Does the investigation and analysis methodology identify the full scope of the accident, including role of management and employees in a way that explains the effects and interdependence of these roles without blame?

Low independence (0) = no independence.
Moderate independence (1) = some independence.
High independence (2) = fully independent.

Acceptability (usage) – usage of technique to date in accident investigations and analyses.

Low acceptability (0) = appears that technique has been developed, but only used as a prototype.
Moderate acceptability (1) = technique has been used in a small number of accident investigation/analyses.
High acceptability (2) = technique has received extensive usage in accident investigations/analyses.

AIMS, CIT and CIM tended to focus on what and how questions, OACM tended to focus more on why questions and RCA more on what, how and why.

All techniques included methodological characteristics that limited consistency, though the level of development of AIMS and OACM might assure moderate levels of consistency. These methods were also expected to be the most comprehensive in the scope of their investigations, along with CIT and RCA, when applied by a skilled investigator. The majority of techniques were felt to be vulnerable to interpretive bias, with RCA and OACM judged most likely to be independent of constraints imposed by more structured techniques.

Error reduction, an important objective in incident investigation, was mostly moderate–high except for OACM, where publications to date have focused only on the application of the method. All techniques benefited from moderate to high levels of auditable documentation and high levels of applicability, but acceptability and usage differed considerably. The latter reflect the fact that contexts in which particular approaches have been developed differ. Less individually intrusive or complex approaches (AIMS, CIM, CIT, SEA) scored high on acceptability, but resource issues will limit the likelihood that particular approaches will be used more widely (CIM, RCA, OACM).

Our assessment does not support any judgement of 'best' methods, as clearly different approaches are more or less suitable for different contexts and purposes. The general point that emerges from this is that developers of techniques and authors of studies and reports that use them need to specify the purpose of the approach and the contexts in which it may be used. AIMS is primarily a high-level reporting system, with wide applicability, and the design of multiple local level systems on the same principle makes little sense. Confidential inquiries are more likely to be sustainable if developed and delivered at regional or national levels. CIT, carried out true to method, also requires significant resources if a large series is to be assembled. On the other hand, SEA, RCA and OACM are primarily aimed at local investigations and analysis, though the potential remains for more formal studies and investigations of series of incidents.

Future challenges

Accident investigation outside health care has acquired a high priority and many industries have invested heavily in the development of proactive and reactive safety assessment tools. Accident investigation methodologies in these settings are generally more clearly defined than those in health care. For example, manuals and descriptions of the methods used are available as well as reports of actual investigations. Health care should now move to adopt the definition and specification of both the process of investigation and techniques employed. Even major investigations, such as those by the Commission for Health Improvement (now the Commission for Health Audit and Inspection) contain very little information on how the investigation was conducted and employ few, if any, of the wide range of techniques available.

Investigation has historically been one of the tasks most difficult to teach because good investigators often have difficulty describing what they do. In recent years all high-risk industries have developed extensive accident investigation training programmes for their employees. Initial courses usually require at least seven days dedicated study, often followed by more advanced and specific training courses at regular intervals thereafter. These organizations recognize that accident investigation is a specialist and complex task, which requires substantial investment in training dedicated accident investigators. Healthcare professionals engaged in investigations are seldom allocated sufficient time, or are relieved of other duties, to enable them to produce a thorough report with serious attention to implementing changes and error reduction strategies. In the long term, however, it may be less expensive, as regards both the human and financial costs, to devote time and resources to investigating incidents to enhance safety and so reduce the overall burden on the healthcare system.

These practical issues should not imply that further development or exploratory use of particular methods in new situations should be discouraged. All methods would benefit from further research on aspects of their performance and especially if methods typically used in one setting are explored in a different speciality or healthcare environment. For example, it is not clear if the characteristics of an AIMS type system will be the same in anaesthetics as in primary care, or whether such a system can be directly imported from another country, where the healthcare staff work in different managerial and legal settings.

Some methods, such as the OACM protocol of Vincent et al. (1999), were originally designed with an individual investigator at the heart of the process. However, this protocol has also been used in other formats, such as structured team discussion and in training and education. Again, the performance of the approach needs to be evaluated when formats and details are modified, as the changes might bring unanticipated problems or benefits that need to be identified by research.

In the course of this work we were struck how SEA in primary care settings was instructive as regards encouraging team interaction and driving change at the clinical level. In our own view this approach might profitably be combined with other techniques, such as OACM or RCA, which are stronger on the analytic frameworks but less so on staff involvement at a local level. What will be needed, however, if such developments are pursued, is a detailed description of the conditions of use and evaluation of the process and outcome of the hybrid approach.

Acknowledgements

The NHS HTA Programme, University College London and Imperial College London funded this work. We are grateful to Professor Charles Vincent for guidance and comment in the conduct of the work. The views and opinions expressed are those of the authors.

Box 10.2 Key points

- There has been little effort to map different approaches to the investigation and analysis of critical incidents in health care.
- Six core techniques are described including background, essential features, theoretical foundations and applications in health care.
- Different approaches have strengths and limitations and are more or less suitable for different contexts and purposes.
- Manuals and protocols for different techniques should be made available and training programmes should be provided so that staff can acquire necessary skills.
- Evaluation research is required to better understand the performance of existing techniques and to explore adaptations, innovations and alternative conditions of use.

References

Amo, M.F. (1998) Root Cause Analysis: a tool for understanding why accidents occur, *Balance*, 2(5): 12–15.

Balcazar, F., Hopkins, B.L. and Suarez, Y. (1985) A critical objective review of performance feedback, *Journal of Organizational Behavior*, 7: 65–89.

Benner, L. (1985) Rating accident models and investigation methodologies, *Journal of Safety Research*, 16: 105–26.

Bennett, I.J. and Danczak, A.F. (1994) Terminal care: improving teamwork in primary care using significant event analysis, *European Journal of Cancer Care*, 3: 54–7.

Berlin, A., Spencer, J.A., Bhopal, R.S. and Zwanenberg, T.D. (1992) Audit of deaths in general practice: pilot study of the critical incident technique, *Quality in Health Care*, 1: 231–5.

Berry, K. and Krizek, B. (2000) Root Cause Analysis in response to a near miss, *Journal for Healthcare Quality*, 22: 16–18.

Beyea, S.C. and Nicoll, L.H. (1999) When an adverse sentinel event is the cause for action, *AORN Journal*, 70: 703–4.

Bradley, C.P. (1992) Uncomfortable prescribing decisions: a critical incident study, *British Medical Journal*, 304: 294–6.

Bucknall, C.E., Slack, R., Godley, C.C., Mackay, T.W. and Wright, S.C. (1999) Scottish Confidential Inquiry into Asthma Deaths (SCIAD), *Thorax*, 54: 978–84.

Burr, M.L., Davies, B.H., Hoare, A., Jones, A., Williamson, I.J. and Holgate, S.K. et al. (1999) A confidential enquiry into asthma deaths in Wales, *Thorax*, 54: 985–9.

Cartlidge, P.H., Jones, H.P., Stewart, J.H., Drayton, M.R., Ferguson, D.S. and Matthes, J.W. et al. (1999) Confidential enquiry into deaths due to prematurity, *Acta Paediatrica*, 88: 220–3.

Chen, P.P., Ma, M., Chan, S. and Oh, T.E. (1998) Incident reporting in acute pain management, *Anaesthesia*, 53: 730–5.

Choy, Y.C., Lee, C.Y. and Inbasegaran, K. (1999) Anaesthesia Incident Monitoring Study in Hospital Kuala Lumpur: the second report, *Medical Journal of Malaysia*, 54: 4–10.

Cooper, J.B., Newbower, R.S. and Kitz, R.J. (1984) An analysis of major errors and equipment failures in anaesthesia management: considerations for prevention and detection, *Anesthesiology*, 60: 34–42.

Cooper, J.B., Newbower, R.A., Long, C.D. and McPeek, B. (1978) Preventable anaesthetic mishaps: a study of human factors, *Anaesthesiology*, 49: 399–406.

Davies, J.M. (2000) Application of the Winnipeg model to obstetric and neonatal audit, *Top Health Information Management*, 20: 12–22.

Drife, J. (1999) Maternal mortality: lessons from the confidential enquiry, *Hospital Medicine*, 60: 156–7.

Durrheim, D.N., Frieremans, S., Kruger, P., Mabuza, A. and de Bruyn, J.C. (1999) Confidential inquiry into malaria deaths, *Bulletin of the World Health Organization*, 77: 263–6.

Eagle, C.J., Davies, J.M. and Reason, J. (1992) Accident analysis of large-scale technological disasters applied to an anaesthetic complication, *Canadian Journal of Anaesthesia*, 39: 118–22.

Flanagan, J.C. (1954) The critical incident technique, *Psychological Bulletin*, 51: 327–58.

Handley, C.C. (2000) Quality improvement through Root Cause Analysis, *Hospital Material Management Quarterly*, 21: 74–8.

Hirsch, K.A. and Wallace, D.T. (1999) Conduct a cost effective RCA by brainstorming, *Hospital Peer Review*, July: 105–22.

JCAHO (2000) Root cause analysis in healthcare: tools and techniques. Oakbrook Terrace, IL: Joint Commission on Accreditation of Healthcare Organizations.

Kirwan, B.I. (1992) Human error identification in human reliability assessment. Part 2: Detailed comparison of techniques. *Applied Ergonomics*, 23: 371–81.

Kluger, M.T. and Short, T.G. (1999) Aspiration during anesthesia: a review of 133 cases from the Australian Anaesthetic Incident Monitoring Study (AIMS), *Anaesthetia*, 54: 19–26.

Morris, G.P. and Morris, R.W. (2000) Anaesthesia and fatigue: an analysis of the first 10 years of the Australian Incident Monitoring Study 1987–1997, *Anaesthesia and Intensive Care*, 28: 300–4.

Payne, J.N., Milner, P.C., Saul, C., Bowns, I.R., Hannay, D.R. and Ramsay, L.E. (1993) Local confidential enquiry into avoidable factors in deaths from strokes and hypertensive disease, *British Medical Journal*, 307: 1027–30.

Pringle, M. (1998) Preventing ischaemic heart disease in one general practice: from one patient, through clinical audit, needs assessment and commissioning into quality improvement, *British Medical Journal*, 317: 1120–3.

Pringle, M., Bradley, C.P., Carmichael, C.M., Wallis, H. and Moore, A. (1995) Significant event auditing: a study of the feasibility and potential of case-based auditing in primary medical care, *Occasional Papers (Royal College of General Practitioners)*, 70: 1–71.

Reason, J. (1997) *Managing the Risks of Organizational Accidents*. Aldershot: Ashgate.

Reason, J.T. (2001) Understanding adverse events: human factors, in C.A. Vincent (ed.) *Clinical Risk Management: Enhancing Patient Safety*. 2nd edn. London: BMJ Publications.

Redpath, L., Stacey, A., Pugh, E. and Holmes, E. (1997) Use of the critical incident technique in primary care in the audit of deaths by suicide, *Quality in Health Care*, 6: 25–8.

Robinson, L.A., Stacy, R., Spencer, J.A. and Bhopal, R.S. (1995) Use of facilitated case discussions for significant event auditing, *British Medical Journal*, 311: 315–18.

Runciman, W.B., Sellen, A., Webb, R.K., Williamson, J.A., Currie, M. and Morgan, C. et al. (1993) The Australian Incident Monitoring: errors, incidents and accidents in anaesthetic practice, *Anaesthesia and Intensive Care*, 21(5): 506–19.

Shinn, J.A. (2000) Root Cause Analysis: a method of addressing errors and patient risk, *Progress in Cardiovascular Nursing*, 15(1): 24–5.

Sinclair, M., Simmons, S. and Cyna, A. (1999) Incidents in obstetric anaesthesia and analgesia: an analysis of 5000 AIMS reports, *Anaesthesia and Intensive Care*, 27: 275–81.

Stanhope, N., Vincent, C.A., Adams, S., O'Connor, A. and Beard, R.W. (1997) Applying human factors methods to clinical risk management in obstetrics, *British Journal of Obstetrics and Gynaecology*, 104: 1225–32.

Steven, D., Malpass, A., Moller, J., Runciman, W.B. and Helps, S.C. (1999) Towards safer drug use in general practice, *Journal of Quality in Clinical Practice*, 19: 47–50.

Vincent, C.A., Adams, S., Hewett, D. and Chapman, J. et al. (1999) *A Protocol for the Investigation and Analysis of Clinical Incidents*. London: Royal Society of Medicine Press Ltd.

Vincent, C.A., Stanhope, N. and Taylor-Adams, S. (2000) Developing a systematic method of analysing serious incidents in mental health, *Journal of Mental Health*, 9: 89–103.

Vincent, C.A., Taylor-Adams, S. and Stanhope, N. (1998) A framework for the analysis of risk and safety in medicine, *British Medical Journal*, 316: 1154–7.

Walker, G.J., Ashley, D.E., McCaw, A.M. and Bernard, G.W. (1986) Maternal mortality in Jamaica, *Lancet*, 1: 486–8.

Waterston, T. (1988) A critical incident study in child health, *Medical Education*, 22: 27–31.

Westcott, R., Sweeney, G. and Stead, J. (2000) Significant event audit in practice: a preliminary study, *Family Practice*, 17: 173–9.

Woloshynowych, M., Rogers, S., Taylor Adams, S. and Vincent, C. (2005) The investigation and analysis of critical incidents in healthcare. NHS HTA Programme.

Wood, B., Catford, J.C. and Cogswell, J.J. (1984) Confidential paediatric inquiry into neonatal deaths in Wessex, 1981 and 1982, *British Medical Journal (Clinical Research Edition)*, 288: 1206–8.

Wright, D., MacKenzie, S.J., Buchan, I., Cairnds, C.S. and Price, L.E. (1991) Critical incidents in the intensive therapy unit, *The Lancet* 338: 676–8.

11

Learning from litigation
The role of claims analysis in patient safety

Charles Vincent, Kieran Walshe, Caroline Davy and Aneez Esmail

One often overlooked source of information on adverse events is the extensive set of data which is collected by healthcare organizations and other agencies on cases of clinical negligence litigation, where patients and their families sue those organizations because they believe they have received negligent care – what we will call here claims data. In the British NHS, organizations like the Medical Defence Union, Medical Protection Society and NHS Litigation Authority collect a large volume of data about cases of clinical negligence, though much of that information is difficult or impossible to access – held in unstructured paper records, distributed across a number of organizations, fragmented across multiple sets of records for the same cases, and not collected consistently using common data definitions and standards. These data have not been collected for the purpose of improvement. They have been gathered primarily by litigation managers, lawyers, risk managers, assessors and others for the purpose of determining legal liability and establishing the quantum of damages. It is information on some of the most serious and damaging errors and adverse events, and an obvious – and increasingly important – question is to what extent this readily available data set on claims might hold important lessons for patient safety, and could be analysed and used to bring about improvements in the quality of health care. Looking to the future, it is equally important to consider whether the way these data are collected and managed in the future might be improved, so as to make data on clinical negligence litigation more directly useful in improving patient safety.

This chapter first places claims data in context as one of a number of ways to study errors and adverse events, and then goes on to review the findings from a number of analyses of claims which have been undertaken in the past two decades. In this section it particularly focuses on the very substantial investment in claims review made by the American Society of Anaesthesiologists since 1984. We then present the findings from recent research undertaken in the British NHS, to examine the potential for using claims data collected by the NHS Litigation Authority, other NHS organizations and the medical defence organizations to improve patient safety. Finally, the chapter draws together from this research the strengths and weaknesses of claims data and claims review, and sets out the circumstances and conditions in which they can be useful and some changes to the way these data are gathered which would improve their utility. The chapter draws extensively on research undertaken for the Department of Health's Patient Safety Research Programme which is reported in full elsewhere (Vincent et al. 2004).

Claims review in context as an approach to detecting errors in patient care

In a comprehensive analysis of approaches to detecting errors in patient care, Thomas and Petersen (2003) noted that there is no perfect way of estimating the incidence of adverse events or of errors. For various reasons, all methods give a partial picture. Record review is comprehensive and systematic, but by definition is restricted to matters noted in the medical record. In contrast, claims are an unrepresentative subset of the totality of errors and adverse events, being biased by specialty, severity and many other factors (Hickson et al. 1994; Vincent et al. 1994). Moreover, different methods are differently oriented towards detecting the incidence of errors and adverse events, active errors and the latent, contributory factors. Thomas and Petersen suggest that the methods can be placed along a continuum with active clinical surveillance of specific types of adverse event (e.g. surgical complications) being the ideal method for assessing incidence, and methods such as claims analysis being more oriented towards exploring the latent conditions for error. Their conclusions about the relative merits and limitations of claims analysis are worth quoting in full:

> Relative to other methods, the strength of claims file analysis lies in its ability to detect latent errors, as opposed to active errors and adverse events. This powerful example of the utility of malpractice claims is balanced by several limitations. Claims are a series of highly selected cases from which it is difficult to generalise. Also, malpractice claims analysis is subject to hindsight bias as well as a variety of other ascertainment and selection biases, and the data present in claims files is not standardised. Finally, although malpractice claims files analysis may identify potential causes of errors and adverse events that may be addressed and studied, the claims files themselves cannot be used to estimate the incidence or prevalence of errors or adverse events or the effect of an intervention to decrease errors and adverse events.
>
> (Thomas and Petersen 2003)

Claims data, as they point out, are not collected in a standardized form and the documents available may be of variable quality. Cases are highly selected and it may be difficult to generalize, though a claims review can produce hypotheses about the causes of problems that may be followed up in more systematic studies. Analysis of claims, indeed, of all events known to have a poor outcome, is also subject to hindsight bias. The term derives from the psychological literature and in particular from experimental studies showing that people exaggerate in retrospect what they knew before an incident occurred – the 'knew it all along' effect. Looking back after the event, the situation faced in actuality by the clinician is inevitably grossly simplified and poorly captured, and the standard of care tends to be judged more harshly in hindsight when the outcome is known to have been wrong (Caplan et al. 1991).

Some key studies of closed claims

We do not offer here a full systematic review of the results of closed claims studies. Rather, our aim is to illustrate the potential and limitations of this method by reviewing some of the major studies. To identify these studies we used our research team's existing knowledge and we searched Medline from 1993 to 2003 using the following search terms: claims analysis, closed claim review, closed claim analysis, medical negligence litigation claims review, insurance claims review and clinical negligence.

Claims data, as Thomas and Petersen have commented, have a number of limitations. However, some important insights have been derived from this approach to studying adverse outcomes. For instance two analyses of British closed claims were carried out in the late 1980s (Ennis and Vincent 1990; Vincent et al. 1991). Cases were drawn from the files of the Medical Protection Society and, for the second study, from the charity Action for Victims of Medical Accidents. The cases considered were births in which the outcome was stillbirth, peri-natal or neonatal death, central nervous system (CNS) damage leading to handicap or maternal death. Junior and middle grade staff were most frequently involved and three major areas of concern were identified: inadequate fetal monitoring, mismanagement of forceps (undue traction, too many attempts), and lack of appropriate involvement of senior staff. Problems included an inability to recognize abnormal or equivocal fetal heart traces and a failure to take appropriate action when an abnormal trace was recognized. Inexperienced doctors were frequently left alone for long periods in labour wards and junior doctors frequently had difficulty in obtaining prompt assistance when problems were recognized.

Vincent (1993) reviewed these and other closed claims studies, and also considered emerging findings from other sources of information about adverse events: occurrence screening (record review), confidential enquiries, critical incident reporting, studies of specific errors and some early observational studies. Many of the studies discussed offered, at that time, only tangential information on patient harm. Claims were one of the most important avenues of enquiry in that they were squarely focused on the issue of harm. Vincent concluded that, whereas claims were not a good reflection of overall risk, valuable information had nevertheless been obtained about underlying clinical problems which, at the very least, provided hypotheses and direction for more focused studies.

The most important series of studies of claims is undoubtedly the ongoing closed claims project of the American Society of Anaesthesiologists (ASA), started in 1984 as part of a number of safety improvement projects, at a time when there was little comprehensive information about the scope and cause of anaesthetic injury (Cheney 1999). In this project a standard report form is completed by an anaesthetic reviewer for every claim where there is enough information to reconstruct the sequence of events and determine the nature and cause of the injury. Typically, a closed claim file consists of the hospital record, the anaesthetic record, narrative statements by the staff involved, statements from the patient, expert and peer reviews and reports of both clinical and legal outcomes. Data entered are subject to further review by project investigators and staff for consistency and completeness before they are assessed as suitable for inclusion in the database. (This careful construction of a customized database is clearly a model for other claims projects.) By 1999, there were more than 4,000 claims in the database. The project has been well reviewed by Cheney (1999) who, looking back over the project's history, considered what had been learned, how the project had affected practice and its potential future role in the light of the emergence of patient safety. We have summarized the principal studies in Table 11.1.

Cheney found that claims were an important source of information on rare events that might not otherwise appear in routine reviews, such as cases of sudden cardiac arrest during spinal anaesthesia (Caplan et al. 1988), and of respiratory problems involving inadequate ventilation, oesophageal intubation and difficult tracheal intubation (Caplan et al. 1990). Whereas all the reports from the database highlight important issues, the authors are assiduous in pointing out the limitations of the database as well as the potential for learning. The principal problems identified in each study are shown in the right-hand column of Table 11.1 and have been summarized by Lee and Domino (2002) (Box 11.1).

Cheney's conclusion about the future of the claims database, in an era of heightened attention to patient safety, is optimistic although hedged with some cautions:

> In summary, the ASA Closed Claims Project is a reporting mechanism that provides an indirect assessment of the safety of anaesthetic practice in the United States. The project represents a national quality assurance system, albeit without a denominator. More than a decade of experience demonstrates that closed claims data can reveal important and previously unappreciated aspects of adverse anaesthetic outcomes. These insights can be used to formulate hypotheses aimed at improving the quality of anaesthetic care, thus providing a tool for advancing patient safety and reducing liability exposure for the anaesthesiologist.

Although anaesthesia-related claims have dominated the research literature, reviews in several other specialties have been carried out. For instance, Neale (1993, 1998a, 1998b) carried out detailed reviews of cases in medical emergencies, in general medicine and in gastroenterology, extracting a number of key lessons to prevent similar outcomes in the future. In the practice of gastroenterology, Neale showed that insufficient attention was paid to the risk:benefit ratio of invasive procedures and to the after-care of patients who suffered an adverse event during a procedure (Neale 1998a).

A particularly sophisticated study of claims was carried out by Gawande and colleagues (2003) who employed a case control design to examine instances of retained instruments and sponges after an operative procedure. By employing this methodology it was possible for Gawande et al. to examine the possible factors that may have led to the error occurring. The main risk factors that predicted the occurrence of a retained foreign body were undergoing emergency surgery, an unplanned change in operation and body mass index (each unit increase of BMI increased risk of retained foreign body). This design overcomes some of the limitations that occur in traditional methods of closed claims analysis, by setting the analysed claims within a representative cohort. However, as is pointed out in the article, there are still limitations to these studies. Not all instances of foreign bodies being left in cavities will result in a claim, and the factors involved in these cases may or may not differ from those that do result in claims.

Table 11.1 Principal studies from the ASA database analysis

Author and paper	Nature of claims and number of cases	Method of case selection	Case review by	Method of analysis	Lessons learned, clinical conclusions	Reflections on claims reviews
Cheney et al. (1994) Burns from warming devices in anesthesia	Claims for burns from 3000 claims in the ASA closed claims database 28 claims	Cases selected from ASA closed claims database for burns from warming devices	Reviewed by anaesthesiologists	Standardized format as employed in other ASA database analyses	Warm IV bags or plastic bottles are a hazard to the patient under anaesthetic, particularly when they are used for purposes other than they are designed for, i.e. maintaining body position instead of providing fluids by IV	As with other ASA database analyses limitations are recognized
Caplan et al. (1997) Adverse Anesthetics Outcomes Arising from Gas Delivery Equipment: A Closed Claims Analysis	3,791 cases in database of the Closed Claims Project 72 claims	Claims associated with gas delivery equipment	Reviewed by practising anaesthetists	Standardized instructions to complete a standardized form detailing patient characteristics, surgical procedures, sequence and location of events, critical incidents, clinical manifestation of injury, standard of care and outcome, preventability of an AE with better monitoring.	The frequency of equipment misuse was 75 per cent compared to only 24 per cent equipment failure suggests human factors are highly significant. Gas delivery equipment failure accounts for between 1–5 per cent of anaesthesia related death and brain damage claims. Claims involving gas delivery equipment account for 2 per cent of the closed claim database.	Claims review limitations include lack of denominator data, no comparison groups, a bias towards adverse outcomes and a reliance on data from direct participants. Reviewer agreement has proved reliable.

Study	Source / claims	Case selection	Review method	Information collected	Findings	Limitations
Cheney et al. (1999) Nerve injury associated with anesthesia: A closed claims analysis	Claims for nerve injury since previous 1990 report, i.e. 1990–1995 670 claims	Cases selected from ASA closed claims database for anaesthetic related nerve injury	Reviewed by practising anaesthesiologists	Standardized information regarding patient characteristics, surgical procedures, sequence and location of events, critical incidents, clinical manifestations of injury, appropriateness of anaesthetic care and outcome	Ulnar neuropathy, the most common anaesthetic related nerve injury (28 per cent). Spinal cord injured most prominent complaint in claims for nerve injury. 16 per cent of claims from ASA project were for anaesthesia related nerve injury	Lack of data regarding total population of risk for injury and non-random retrospective data collection. No information regarding total number of anaesthetics provided or specialization versus general anaesthetic split.
Domino et al. (1999b) Awareness during Anesthesia: A closed claims analysis	Drawn from a total of 4,183 claims from the database of the American Society of Anesthetists (ASA) Closed Claim Project collected between 1961 and 1995. 79 claims	Claims that involved awareness during anaesthesia	Reviewers not specified but given specific instructions about how to use a standardized review form.	Information on patient characteristics, surgical procedures, sequence and location of events, critical incidents, clinical manifestations of injury, standard of care and outcome. Severity of injury score was grouped into temporary/non-disabling injury or disabling/permanent/death	Claims for women involved a lower severity of injury than those for men suggesting that women may be more likely to file a claim for awareness during anaesthesia. Claims for recall during GA only accounted for 1.5 per cent of the claims on the ASA database. 87 per cent of claims are from elective surgery patients.	Closure of an awareness during anaesthesia claim may be quicker than in more severe claims thus making a greater proportion of these types of claims in the database.

Continued overleaf

Table 11.1 (Continued)

Author and paper	Nature of claims and number of cases	Method of case selection	Case review by	Method of analysis	Lessons learned, clinical conclusions	Reflections on claims reviews
Domino et al. (1999a) Airway injury during anesthesia: a closed claim analysis	Airway injury claims taken from the American society of Anesthesiologists closed claims project database 266 claims	Airway injury cases from anaesthetic database	Reviewers not specified but given specific instructions about how to use a standardized review form.	Information on patient characteristics, surgical procedures, sequence and location of events, critical incidents, clinical manifestations of injury, standard of care and outcome. Severity of injury was grouped into temporary/ non-disabling injury or disabling/ permanent/ death	A higher proportion of airway injury claims involved females, elective procedures and outpatient procedures. Difficult intubation was a factor in 39 per cent of airway injury cases compared to 9 per cent of general anaesthetic claims	Inability of closed claim analysis to provide estimate of risk because no denominator data. No comparison groups probably bias towards adverse outcomes reliance on direct participants rather than impartial observer

| Lee and Domino (2002) The Closed Claim Project: Has it influenced anesthetic practice and outcome? | Closed claims for adverse outcomes in anaesthetics between 1961 and 1999. Data obtained from 35 liability insurance companies. Dental claims excluded 5,480 claims | Data collected from cases where there was sufficient information to understand what had happened and to judge nature and causation of injury. | Trained reviewers who are practising anaesthetists | Trained anaesthetists used a standardized form to collate specified information particularly assessing the appropriateness of anaesthetic care. Each claim was also assigned a severity of injury score. The reviewer made a summary of the case and all data was sent to a Closed Claim Project Committee where at least two practising anaesthetists reviewed the claim. Claims were then classified into groupings for analysis. |

Table 11.1 *(Continued)*

Author and paper	Nature of claims and number of cases	Method of case selection	Case review by	Method of analysis	Lessons learned, clinical conclusions	Reflections on claims reviews
Ross (2003) ASA closed claims in obstetrics: lessons learned (Reanalysis of an earlier paper by Chadwick H S. (1996)	5,300 cases from the Closed Claims database. 635 (12 per cent) associated with obstetrical anaesthetic cases	Obstetric anaesthetic cases from the ASA Closed Claims database	As above	As above	Mostly supports commonly held views about the risks of obstetric anaesthesia but highlights the fact that minor injuries are more common in obstetric files than non-obstetric files. Suggestions for avoiding malpractice claims in obstetrics include: careful personal conduct, establishing good rapport, involvement in prenatal education, early pre-anaesthetic evaluation, providing realistic expectations, regularly reviewing potential major and minor risks	Unfortunately, the claims data does not give general incidence figures for adverse events and anaesthetists may be named in a claim where there was no anaesthetic-related adverse event. Also claims reflect out of date practice because of the time lapse between opening and closing a claim. But they do allow the identification of common injuries, the nature of precipitating events and differences between regional and general anaesthetics

---

Box 11.1 Limitations of anaesthesia closed claims analysis

1. Subset of adverse outcomes:

   (a) Few adverse outcomes end in claims.
   (b) Bias towards more severe injuries.

2. Inability to calculate incidence:

   (a) Lack of denominator data.
   (b) Geographic imbalance.

3. Other sources of bias:

   (a) Changes in practice patterns.
   (b) Partial reliance on direct participants.
   (c) Retrospective transcription of data.
   (d) Absence of rigorous comparison groups.
   (e) Low reliability of judgements of appropriateness of care.
   (f) Outcome bias.

Source: Lee and Domino (2002)

Analysing claims in four specialties in the NHS

In recent research commissioned by the Department of Health in the United Kingdom to explore the value of claims data in improving patient safety in the NHS, four specialty reviews were carried out spanning medicine and surgery, obstetrics, primary care and mental health (Vincent et al. 2004). Cases were selected from a number of different databases, depending on the availability of the relevant data in each of the various sources. Four experienced clinicians, each with both medico-legal and research experience, reviewed samples of cases from each of the four specialty areas. Each reviewer identified one or more themes (such as suicide in mental health patients), which was of both clinical and medico-legal importance. Reviewers were asked to focus on the clinical issues and potential for learning clinical lessons, but also to reflect on the value of the process of claims review and to note difficulties encountered with data quality, coding or the review process as they went.

Readers should consult the full report for a description of the methodology of the review and details of the clinical lessons of claims review in each specialty. In this chapter we draw on the principal conclusions of the individual studies to examine the more general question of the value of claims review.

Only a proportion of cases available were suitable for full review. Those for medicine and surgery were pre-selected to some extent, but only about 70 per cent of the remainder had sufficient data for full review. In addition, an average of ten years had elapsed between the occurrence of the original incident and our review, slightly less for medicine and surgery. The amount of paperwork to be reviewed for each case varied greatly. Documents included expert reports for each case, witness statements, legal summaries, and other documentation, such as coroners' reports and statements of claim. An average of 4.7 documents were reviewed per case, with the number varying between 0 and 19.

Even in the restricted set of claims files that have sufficient data for review, reviewers judged that there was a number of cases in which the injury sustained was not caused by medical management. Injury was judged to be due to the disease process in 20 per cent of cases overall, and in an additional 16 per cent of cases reviewers were unable to make any firm assessment of causation of injury. However, reviewers were generally able to make judgements about the nature of the principal clinical issue identified, in the sense of pinpointing a failure in diagnosis, a failure to monitor, problems with drugs or fluids, and so on.

Clinical issues are fully discussed within the specialty reports. In Box 11.2 we have summarized some of the main themes in order to address the general question of

---

Box 11.2 Clinical lessons learned from claims reviews

Surgery and general medicine

- A full history and clinical examination remains vital to the art of diagnosis.
- There is a need for proper assessment of all the evidence at time of discharge and clear guidelines to GPs and to clinical staff in follow-up clinics.
- It is necessary to maintain awareness both of diseases that are less common than they used to be (e.g. perforated peptic ulcers) and common diseases of the past that are reappearing (e.g. tuberculosis).
- SHO/Registrars should not be taking full responsibility for assessment of patients in outpatient clinics.
- Emergency resuscitation equipment needs to be available, in working order and staff trained to use it.

General practice

- Computerized decision aids may assist diagnosis of rare diseases such as diabetes in children.
- Robust systems of care for the ongoing management of diabetes in adults are vital.
- Primary care trusts need to be able to access information about rare diseases easily.
- Lack of knowledge was a contributory factor in many of the cases analysed.

Obstetrics

- Further training in CTG interpretation may be beneficial in avoiding adverse events, to ensure correct use of these monitors.
- Failure to adhere to guidelines may be an important cause of adverse events.
- Problems within the system of care, with doctor–patient relationships and with teamwork/supervision were noted.
- Whereas many of the adverse events involved more junior staff, the judgements of the consultants/midwives were also questionable on occasion.

Mental health

- Observation of patients on section needs to be defined in care plans.
- Psychiatric referral needs to be more easily accessed so that at risk patients can be seen quickly.
- Nursing notes need to be amalgamated into medical notes so that a full assessment can be made including a list of observations, past history, current stresses and symptoms.
- More and better training needs to be put in place for diagnosis.

whether clinical lessons of importance can be identified from claims review. These comments were drawn both from the reports themselves and from reviewers' case summaries and additional comments. While reviewers, drawing on their own experience, are clearly inferring more general clinical problems from a small set of cases, they nevertheless consider that these cases do draw attention to important clinical issues.

In our review, we specifically asked reviewers to comment on a defined list of contributory factors (Vincent et al. 1998). Since 40 per cent of cases were reported as having contributory team factors to the injury/claim, clearly teamworking is a significant problem. The skills and behaviour of individual clinicians were judged to have contributed to the problem in 17 per cent of cases and task factors accounted for 23 per cent of cases. Organizational/management issues were found in 25 per cent of cases and work environment factors were judged the least frequent contributory factor at 6 per cent, but these may of course simply be harder to discern or infer from medical records and claims data. Some factors were particularly relevant to specific specialties, e.g. patient characteristics were judged to be contributory in 92 per cent of mental health cases and 49 per cent of primary care cases. However, we should caution that reviewers were very often 'unable to judge' whether a particular factor had any bearing on the case in question.

Reviewers felt confident in drawing important clinical lessons from at least a proportion of cases, and were often aided by the high quality of expert reports. However, they also noted a number of limitations of the claims review process which are summarized in Box 11.3.

The scope and value of claims review

It is worth restating the obvious but important point that claims data have not been collected for the purpose of improving clinical care or contributing to patient safety. The analysis of claims data does of course shed light on patterns of litigation and the specific characteristics of cases that have come to litigation. However, almost all the studies reviewed here have stressed that claims are an unrepresentative sample of adverse outcomes of health care and represent only a very small proportion of instances in which care has been sub-standard or patients have come to some harm. A host of factors affect whether or not a patient sues, with communication and doctor–patient relationship a major predictor of litigation (Hickson et al. 1994; Vincent et al. 1994). Just as claims databases were not developed to enhance patient safety but to manage claims, the same is true of expert reports. Their purpose is to assist the

---

Box 11.3 Limitations of the process of claims review, the UK experience

Evidence

- Full case notes sometimes required for detailed assessment.
- Inadequate clinical notes impede the whole process.
- There is a very variable quality of evidence.

Organization of evidence

- Expert witness reports and internal enquiry report may be missing from case files.
- Files are established for documenting a legal process, not for the purposes of study, therefore not all information that may have been required was available.
- Clear marking of where reports, statements and letters are to be found would help, especially in multiple file cases.

Timescale

- Delay between closing of case and claims analysis, so changes may have occurred in working practice.
- If investigated, documented and analysed at the time of incident, instead after a number of years, many of the shortcomings of this method would be overcome.

Dropped/withdrawn claims

- Notes on reasons why claim is not pursued would be useful.
- Death of patient inevitably means claim is dropped.
- Sometimes claim is withdrawn although care is clearly below standard.
- Where cases are barred because of statute (time) limitations, important lessons are lost.
- Sometimes causality may not be proved but nonetheless lessons could be learned from these cases.

---

adjudication of a case. However, in the course of this analysis the expert reviewer, whether appointed by the plaintiff or defendant, will comment on the nature of the sub-standard care and may, by chance if not design, comment on background factors that contributed to the sub-standard care. A good expert report can be a very illuminating document.

In spite of these inherent limitations, the authors of our own reviews, and of other studies of claims, were all able to draw conclusions about problems in the process of care in the cases they reviewed. Not all cases are suitable for review and they vary considerably in the amount of detail and extent to which lessons can be learned. In general, however, clinical themes are apparent, in terms of defined problems at particular phases of the care process and, to some extent, in the detection of background, contributory factors. To achieve this, reviewers have to draw extensively on their own clinical experience. Their reviews, and it is no disrespect to say this, are more a matter of interpretation than data collection. Reviewers, and the experts who reviewed the original notes, are often reading beyond the information available to surmise what must have happened to produce this outcome.

The methodological limitations of claims review have been well summarized by the ASA reviewers (Box 11.1). They include the lack of denominator data, bias towards more severe injuries, problems in the reliability of judgements, outcome and hindsight bias, the unrepresentative nature of claims, and so on. The most important point to make here is that these conclusions have been echoed by many other reviewers of claims and by our own specialty reviewers (Box 11.3).

In addition to problems inherent in the claims review process, our reviewers were also very concerned about the completeness of the record and the quality of the data available. Clinical notes, where available, were of varying quality as were expert reports and other documents. Key information was sometimes missing and on occasion the reviewer felt unable to make an assessment from the expert reports alone, and would ideally have needed to see the full medical record. Organization and retrieval of data were sometimes difficult. Some of these problems are potentially remediable. It is noteworthy that the ASA closed claims project invests considerable time and resources to ensuring that full clinical records are retrieved whenever possible, documents and facts are checked and all possible material retrieved before a case is entered in a database. With sufficient resources, this could also be done in the UK. However, inevitably, claims that do not proceed or are withdrawn will often have insufficient data for review and it may not always be possible to assemble a defined set of documents that might be considered a 'minimum data set' for claims review.

Future challenges

Claims review is only one of a number of approaches to the study of adverse events, and other methods of enquiry (all of which have their own limitations) do not suffer from some of the major disadvantages of claims review. Systematic record review captures incidence much more effectively. Claims data do have the ability, when data quality are good, to capture important facts about the quality of care and factors contributing to adverse events. But contributory factors can be much more effectively assessed by contemporaneous interviews and observation (Vincent et al. 2000; Vincent et al. 2004) than by screening medical records and reports several years after the event. Studies of any kind which prospectively set out to capture some aspect of errors and adverse events can define data collection methods and data quality in a way that opportunistic, retrospective review of claims data never can. In general, we would suggest, a better understanding of incidents can be achieved if investigations begin soon after the incident has occurred.

Claims review, then, is unlikely to be the method of choice for assessing either the incidence of or understanding of adverse outcomes. But are there any circumstances in which claims data could provide insights not available by other methods? Here again, the ASA closed claims project provides a model, in that the great strength of claims data is that they can provide information on rare events, not easily detectable by routine review or observation. Large-scale reporting systems, such as that of the National Patient Safety Agency or the Australian Incident Monitoring System, also have this advantage but it is possible that claims could provide additional information or detect other types of incident.

Defining a minimum data set for the review of a set of claims would allow some standardization of the process as well as ensuring that, at least for those cases of interest, all relevant documents were assembled. While this might not always be necessary from the legal point of view, it would be enormously helpful from the point of view of learning from claims. Assembling a standard set of documents would also be a first step to standardization of the process and some basic quality control in at least ensuring that all necessary papers had been collated. Case review of individual claims, by its very nature, cannot be a completely standardized process. Nevertheless, it would certainly be possible to enhance the quality of the information available by, for instance, devising a standard set of questions that expert reports should address. While lawyers do attempt, in many cases, to do this, their instructions are probably too generic in a research context. If particular clinical issues had been identified for claims review, experts could easily append answers to a standard set of questions at the time of compiling a report. As they would be reviewing the records anyway, this would not be costly. Alternatively, clinical reviewers could simply use the basic medical records and answer the questions themselves, as we have done. Whatever system is adopted, the main point is that a defined set of questions aimed at specific clinical and organizational issues will produce more robust and persuasive analyses than an unstructured *post hoc* review.

In summary, then, we would propose that claims review can be useful as an approach to the understanding of error and adverse outcomes. The strength of claims review lies in its potential to provide rich information and comment on particular cases, with the caution that these may not be representative of the wider class of adverse outcomes. However, a number of preconditions have to be met:

- That either the condition under investigation is sufficiently rare not to be easily detectable by other means or claims data offer additional information not otherwise available.

- Other methods of investigating this class of problem have been assessed and claims review has been found to provide additional information of value.

- That cases are selected and analysed as soon as possible after the incident has occurred.

- That a better attempt is made to understand the patient's perspective and experience as this is, potentially, a strength of claims data in comparison to other methods.

- That due consideration is given, where possible, to defining an appropriate control group (Gawande et al. 2003).

- Claims data are assembled in a central database and are checked and subject to quality control at the time of entry to the database (as with the ASA closed claims analysis).

- The results of claims review are treated as working hypotheses and subject to further investigation in more formal studies.

- The claims review is used only as part of a more general quality and safety improvement strategy.

- Expert claims reviewers work to a defined data collection template and a defined set of questions.

These criteria make it clear that there is now no case for an *ad hoc* claims review that relies on claims data that have been assembled for legal purposes only and with no thought to their use in improving the quality and safety of patient care. Other sources of data and approaches are now increasingly available which mean that form of claims review is probably unhelpful. However, we believe that there are circumstances in which claims review can be justified as a valuable approach to a problem in health care.

Acknowledgements

Thanks to Graham Neale, Max Elstein and Jenny Firth Cozens who undertook the specialty based reviews referred to in this chapter, and to Paul Fenn and Alistair Gray who led the quantitative analysis of the claims review data.

Box 11.4 Key points

- An extensive set of data is collected in healthcare organizations and other agencies on cases of clinical negligence litigation – when patients and their families sue those organizations because they believe they have received negligent care.
- Claims data are not collected for the purposes of improving patient safety or the quality of care, and they are often held in unstructured paper records, distributed across organizations, not collected consistently using common definitions and standards and only available some considerable time after the episode of care to which they refer.
- There have been many past analyses of claims which have produced important and clinically relevant findings and have contributed to improvements in safety and quality.
- Recent research in the British NHS has tested the value of claims data held by the NHS Litigation Authority and the medical defence organizations, and identified a series of important clinical issues.
- If claims data were collected by the agencies involved in a more structured and standardized format, and held in forms which are more readily manageable, then the considerable investment made in collecting such data for the primary purpose of managing clinical negligence litigation could yield greater benefits for patient safety.
- Other mechanisms for analysing errors and adverse events are likely to be more timely, complete and accurate than claims review, which suffers from significant biases and limitations, but there will still be circumstances where claims review can make an important and distinctive contribution.

References

Caplan, R.A., Posner, K. and Cheney, F. (1991) Effect of outcome on physician judgements of appropriateness of care, *Journal of the American Medical Association*, 266: 793–4.

Caplan, R.A., Posner, K., Ward, R. and Cheney, F. (1990) Adverse respiratory events in anesthesia, *Anesthesiology*, 72: 828–33.

Caplan, R.A., Ward, R.J., Posner, K. and Cheney, F.W. (1988) Unexpected cardiac arrest during spinal anesthesia: a closed claims analysis of predisposing factors, *Anesthesiology*, 68: 5–11.

Cheney, F. (1999) The American Society of Anesthesiologists Closed Claims Project: what we have learned, how has it affected practice, and how will it affect practice in the future, *Anesthesiology*, 91: 552–6.

Ennis, M. and Vincent, C.A. (1990) Obstetric accidents: a review of 64 cases, *British Medical Journal*, 300: 1365–7.

Gawande, A., Studdert, D., Orav, E., Brennan, T.A. and Zinner, M. (2003) Risk factors for retained instruments and sponges after surgery, *New England Journal of Medicine*, 348: 229–35.

Hickson, G.B., Clayton, E.W., Entman, S.S., Miller, C.S., Githens, P.B., Whetten-Goldstein, K. and Sloan, F.A. (1994) Obstetricians' prior malpractice experience and patients' satisfaction with care, *Journal of the American Medical Association*, 272: 1583–7.

Lee, L. and Domino, K. (2002) The closed claims project: has it influenced anesthetic practice and outcome?, *Anesthesiology Clinics of North America*, 20: 485–501.

Neale, G. (1993) Clinical analysis of 100 medicolegal cases, *British Medical Journal*, 307: 1483–7.

Neale, G. (1998a) Reducing risks in gastroenterological practice, *Gut*, 42: 139–42.

Neale, G. (1998b) Risk management in the care of medical emergencies after referral to hospital, *Journal of the Royal College of Physicians of London*, 32: 125–9.

Thomas, E.J. and Petersen, L.A. (2003) Measuring errors and adverse events in health care, *Journal of General Internal Medicine*, 18: 61–7.

Vincent, C.A. (1993) The study of errors and accidents in medicine, in C.A. Vincent, M. Ennis and R.J. Audley (eds) *Medical Accidents*. Oxford: Oxford University Press, pp. 17–33.

Vincent, C.A., Davy, C., Esmail, A., Neale, G., Elstein, M., Firth Cozens, J. and Walshe, K. (2004) *Learning from Litigation: An Analysis of Claims for Clinical Negligence*. Manchester: University of Manchester, Manchester Centre for Healthcare Management.

Vincent, C.A., Martin, T. and Ennis, M. (1991) Obstetric accidents: the patient's perspective, *British Journal of Obstetrics and Gynaecology*, 98: 390–5.

Vincent, C., Taylor-Adams, S., Chapman, E.J., Hewett, D., Prior, S., Strange, P. and Tizzard, A. (2000) How to investigate and analyse clinical incidents: clinical risk unit and association of litigation and risk management protocol, *British Medical Journal*, 320: 777–81.

Vincent, C.A., Taylor-Adams, S. and Stanhope, N. (1998) Framework for analysing risk and safety in clinical medicine, *British Medical Journal*, 316: 1154–7.

Vincent, C.A., Young, M. and Phillips, A. (1994) Why do people sue doctors? A study of patients and relatives taking legal action, *Lancet*, 343: 1609–13.

12

Ethnographic methods in patient safety

Rachael Finn and Justin Waring

The ethnographic contribution to patient safety research

This chapter explores the contribution of ethnographic methodologies and methods to patient safety research. Notwithstanding methodological debate and disagreement, ethnography is typically associated with the in-depth, inductive exploration of the social world through the use of highly contextualized and detailed methods that centre on the interpretation of shared meanings, actions, processes and institutions with a given social and cultural context (Hammersley and Atkinson 1995). Although 'culture' remains a highly debated concept, as a shared set of deeply held beliefs, assumptions or way of viewing the world, it is an integral and pervasive feature of healthcare organization and delivery (Dingwall and Finn 2000). Furthermore, the relationship between culture and safety has been firmly established in safety management literature (e.g. Reason 1997; Helmreich and Merritt 1998), and the creation of a 'safety culture' has been designated as the first of seven steps to 'patient safety' (NPSA 2003). Although there are several measures and tools to quantify and classify 'safety cultures' or 'climates' and there are several observational studies that claim to 'be' ethnographies, there is little consideration of what ethnography involves or, more importantly, what it can offer to patient safety research in terms of a deep, holistic and contextualized account of social cultures.

This chapter proceeds with a review of the methodological foundations of ethnography and shows how these translate into research methods. It is important to note that many more detailed and sophisticated texts accomplish this task and therefore the intention here is to provide a brief account of its underlying principles and how it is practised 'in the field'. The chapter then illustrates the contribution of ethnography to patient safety research through drawing on existing examples of ethnographic research that explore the important socio-cultural facets of healthcare delivery that are relevant to current issues of patient safety. It is anticipated that this chapter will clarify and promote the use of ethnography in patient safety research and illustrate its relationships with other theoretical perspectives and methodologies.

Principles of ethnography

Ethnography is a particular perspective to social scientific inquiry. It incorporates a *methodology*, or set of assumptions concerning the nature of the social world (ontology) and how we can research it (epistemology), and a set of *methods* or tools by which to access or capture that world. Ethnography has a clear affinity with the study of culture, with the intention of making explicit and interpreting the historical and relatively taken-for-granted and shared meanings, values and actions that underpin social action. Fundamentally, this reflects the roots of ethnography in *naturalist* methodology, the assumptions of which define the very nature of questions asked about the social world and how we can go about addressing these.

Naturalism grew out of an increasing attack upon positivism during the 1960s, and at the level of ontology challenges the assumption that there is an objective social world reducible to that externally observed by the researcher. Naturalism argues that the social world is socially constructed – actively created and recreated through the ongoing interpretations and responses of social actors in specific contexts (Berger and Luckman 1967). Essentially, the focus of research becomes 'the way in which different people experience, interpret and structure their lives' (Burgess 1984: 3). If we are to understand social action, we need to understand and access the meanings and interpretations of the world that underlie and guide it (Hammersley and Atkinson 1995). The social world is studied as it naturally occurs, independent of scientific manipulation. A rich understanding of activities and meanings is gained from 'the inside' through direct participation in an inductive, grounded way.

The central objective of ethnography is, therefore, to understand the social meaning given to objects, actions, and events and how they reflect, reiterate and renegotiate wider social discourses and cultures. Here meaning is not conceptualized as universal or static but it is seen as contextualized, negotiated and sustained within relative sociocultural and historical settings. How people perceive, interpret and make sense of something is shaped by the norms, practices and knowledge(s) within which they engage. Through talking with individuals and studying social interaction, ethnographic research has the potential to explore how meanings relate and contribute to a given social setting. Furthermore, ethnography is concerned with understanding how meanings are 'learned', shared and can reinforce social cohesion and togetherness; or alternatively, represent a source of disunity and deviance. In the context of occupational and organizational work, a collective way of thinking and behaving is important for not only informing social practice but also for maintaining a sense of identity and meaning in work. Ethnographic research has the potential to explore the processes through which individual members are socialized into a culture and come to acquire collective beliefs, while understanding how collective attitudes inform behaviour and relate to wider social, organizational and occupational structures. This means that ethnographic research is typically in-depth and small scale, capturing the complexity and richness of social world from the perspectives of those who make up the social setting.

What implications do these methodological assumptions carry for researching culture and patient safety? Ultimately, they represent a shift beyond survey instruments commonly employed to capture the 'subjectivity' of healthcare contexts and highlight a distinction between 'culture' and 'climate'. Culture is deeply embedded in social practice, a set of collective, taken-for-granted, tacit assumptions and beliefs that are hard to explicitly articulate but come into play in the course of micro-social interaction. Culture guides collective social action in specific contexts and situations in everyday work and cannot be divorced from that. Thus, it can be distinguished as something deeper and different from individual attitudes or beliefs towards a set of statements relating to safety explored by survey instruments. These tools examine 'climate' removed from context and practice, investigating correlations with organizational and performance variables *post hoc*. They do not capture how deeper assumptions emerge and influence collective work practices in specific, localized situations and contextual conditions. This requires getting close to the everyday working practices of healthcare professionals by participation in natural settings, an approach at the heart of the ethnographic perspective. In this way, cultural assumptions and their relationship to specific organizational conditions and practices pertaining to safety can be revealed.

Ethnography in practice

This section gives a brief overview of the main methods and issues of ethnographic research (for a detailed discussion, see Burgess 1984; Hammersley and Atkinson 1995; Brewer 2000). In selecting specific methods, the ethnographer is a 'methodological pragmatist' (Schatzman and Strauss 1973), choosing those that best address the particular research question in hand. Thus, while observation is the primary ethnographic method, triangulation – or the use of multiple methods – is common.

However, conducting ethnography is not just the application of a set of methods and rules, but a *process* requiring judgement in context (Hammersley and Atkinson 1995). Ethnography is inductive, therefore inherently flexible and developmental, requiring the researcher to continually monitor and modify the research process and their role within it as they interact with that social world. As Burgess (1984: 6) states, 'field research is concerned with research processes as well as research methods'. This means that fundamental aspects of research design, such as sampling, access and methods, are constantly revisited and developed. Described here are some of the common methods of carrying out ethnographic research.

Participant observation

Observations are the core method of ethnography. They enable the researcher to gain detailed insight into the social world through witnessing or directly engaging in social activities. This participation enables the researcher to experience and 'see' the world from the perspective of social actors, learning their language, systems of meanings, and exploring the symbolic and cultural significance of rituals and routines that make up everyday life. Thus, observation not only includes watching what happens but also listening to conversations, carrying out informal interviews and collecting documents as the researcher participates in daily life. This immersion enables the production of a rich, 'thick description' (Geertz 1973) of the setting. Conducting ethnographic observations is time-consuming and requires substantial contact with the social setting to the point where the researcher becomes a 'fixture' and has access to the detail minutiae of social practice. The researcher role can vary both between and within studies, along the continuum from 'complete observer' to 'complete participant' and in terms of the degree of familiarity with the setting being studied. The aim is always to make the 'strange familiar' and the 'familiar strange', to balance 'getting close' without 'going native' (Gold 1969).

The focus of the observations will obviously vary according to the setting being studied, the questions being asked and the underlying theoretical orientation of the research. However, it is often common for ethnographic research to study the norms and customs that make up social action and interaction, or the routines, rituals and ceremonies that make up social practice. For health service research, this could include the customary features of doctor–patient interactions, the conventions of professional teamwork, the rituals of hand washing, or the routines of the ward round. Ethnographic observations involve more than merely describing these events, but through participating and sharing in these events the aim is to understand why they occur as they do, what meanings they hold for participants and what underlying cultural significance they have for those who take part, both explicitly and implicitly. In doing so, the researcher is able to elaborate the cultural significance of these actions and interactions, such as the way doctor–patient consultations serve as an expression of power or authority, or how rituals of nursing reinforce professional identity and social order. In terms of patient safety, ethnographic observations can explore how the norms and rituals of professional practice can have potentially latent consequences for safety. For example, the dominance and authority of the doctor can make it difficult for other professional groups to 'speak out' and identify potential risks to safety, or the collegial norms of professional membership foster an exclusionary approach to safety and inhibit participation in incident reporting.

Participant observation can be challenging, since the researcher is not only involved in data collection, but also in an ongoing negotiation of access, sampling and establishing relationships with actors in complex social settings. For this reason, the use of 'key informants' by ethnographers is common; these are selected 'insider' participants who aid the researcher in orientating to the setting, developing relationships and gaining access to others. The researcher, however, needs to select carefully, as the roles and relationships of key informants in that setting can impact upon the success in gaining access to and trust of other participants.

Interviews

Interviews are a central method employed in ethnography. A distinction can be made between short and informal interviews or 'chats' conducted during the course of observations and more structured and formal interviews conducted typically outside of the immediate social setting. The former are particularly useful for clarifying issues or querying a given social event, while the latter often take a broader perspective and ask potentially more personal or biographical questions. In 'true' ethnography, interviews are used in conjunction with participant observation to build upon the knowledge and rapport established and to follow up what has been observed and give access to situations not directly witnessed or inaccessible (Brewer 2000). However, 'ethnographic style' interviews can be used as a stand-alone qualitative technique, where access or research questions are not suited to observational methods.

Regardless of the style of interview used, ethnographic interviews can be described as 'conversations with a purpose' (Burgess 1984: 102), capturing the conversational style of interviewing, where emphasis is placed upon the use of open-ended questions to prioritize respondents' views over those of the researcher around a set of research questions and themes. Respondents talk freely in their own terms to express their understandings and explore meanings to produce data in rich, natural language. They provide the researcher with the opportunity to further explore observational findings and to probe the beliefs, views and assumptions of participants. The focus of the interview and the questions asked will vary according to the aims of the study and theoretical context, but a common aim is to acquire narrative accounts of the social world, to explore how individuals make sense and give meaning to their world, and to understand how their beliefs, assumptions, values and meanings relate to how they act and interact with others. For patient safety research, ethnographic interviews could involve, for example, asking professionals to describe their work in detail, identifying what they regard to be the threats to safety, or more implicitly examining norms, assumptions and beliefs around issues pertaining to safety. These accounts, narratives and descriptions can be explored to understand the underlying beliefs and assumptions about what are the underlying causes of patient harm, how blame and responsibility are apportioned and what they believe should be done to improve safety. Again, depending on the focus of the study, this information can be telling about how individuals see themselves as professionals, how they think about their colleagues or the organization they work in and how they try to maintain notions of competence, identify and trust.

Documentary evidence

Documentary evidence is a valuable source of ethnographic data. Social institutions produce a range of documentation as part of their everyday, routine functioning. These can provide insight into the organization and subjectivity of social life, revealing the social processes and social categories within a particular setting. While one advantage of documents is that they are often naturally occurring, ethnographers sometimes solicit their production for the purposes of a research project (e.g. through diaries).

Documentary evidence consists of such things as organizational charts, process information, memos, material artefacts, diaries, records and autobiographies. Documentary evidence can be classified, making distinctions between those that are pre-existing or produced for the purposes of research. It is also possible to distinguish between 'official', personal, public or private, contemporary or historical and primary or secondary documentary sources. For patient safety research, there are numerous sources of documentary data, such as patient records, incident reports, risk scores or action plans. For ethnographic research it is important to consider, however, that documentary sources can be analysed in various ways, for example, taken on 'face value' as descriptive accounts of the social setting, or analysed for their underlying cultural and discursive features, seeking out the implicit assumptions and cultural preferences related to patient safety. For example, the contents of an incident report would not necessarily be treated as a given 'truth' but would be seen as a particular subjective interpretation and expression of a patient safety incident that implicitly reflects the wider cultural context of the author and contains underlying assumptions about how improved safety should be achieved. However documents are employed, the researcher needs to consider their authenticity, source, purpose and availability as they occur within the social setting, and should have a strategy for sampling from those available.

Ethnographic studies of medical culture and safety

The chapter now turns to briefly illustrating the contributions of ethnography to patient safety research. Many studies have explored the socio-cultural context of healthcare organization and delivery, and professional work and culture in health care. Accordingly, there are numerous implicit and explicit ethnographic works relevant to issues of safety. Three themes have been selected here to more thoroughly explore the cultural context of patient safety: (1) how issues of safety are given meaning; (2) how collegial cultures inform practices of safety; and (3) how professional teamwork cultures contextualize safety.

Social meanings of error and safety

There are a number of works that directly or indirectly engage with the social meaning of error in medical work, which relate meaning to the lived experience of medical practice (Paget 2004), the uncertainties of medical knowledge (Rosenthal 1995; Fox 2000) or the maintenance of professional status (Freidson 1975). Perhaps the best-known work in this area is Charles Bosk's (1979) *Forgive and Remember*, which examines the social meaning of error in the context of surgical training. His ethnographic study involved participant observations of surgical training and through his work he shows that the meaning of error is constructed through the relationship between trainees and their supervising 'attendings'. In his analysis he categorizes the different ways in which medical errors are interpreted and given meaning. What he describes as *judgement errors* relate to evaluations of diagnosis and decision-making by trainees and the extent to which these conferred with the experiences and expectations of the attending. Similarly, *technical errors* relate to meeting the procedural expectations of surgical practice and performance. *Normative errors* referred less to the technical activities of surgical care but were associated with the conduct and personal behaviour of a trainee, such as a poor bedside manner, failure to communicate problems to superiors or conduct unbecoming to a surgeon.

Importantly, in identifying the different social meanings of error, Bosk was able to explore how social meaning corresponds with the socialization processes of surgical training and the way in which mistakes are controlled through social practice.

Specifically, judgement and technical errors were seen as inevitable aspects of surgical training that could be beneficial in identifying future training requirements.

Bosk suggests that the philosophy behind surgical training is to encourage trainees to gain clinical experience without excessive supervision; mistakes are therefore a 'regrettable but inevitable part of the baptism under fire that is house officer training' (Bosk 1986: 466). However, normative errors were less likely to be forgiven and served to reveal something more fundamental about the trainees' appropriateness for the surgical profession. Bosk's work therefore shows how the meaning of error is socially located, in this case within the context of surgical training, and importantly how these culturally relative meanings serve to inform subsequent social action.

Meanings are a constituent part and emergent feature of a culture and are central to informing social practice. Within the current 'patient safety', it therefore becomes important to appreciate that our definitions and understanding of error or adverse event are not universal or objective but reflect prevailing theoretical and cultural assumptions, for example, about good and bad performance. Furthermore, how such incidents are given meaning by one social group may not be shared by others and therefore the expectations of incident reporting may vary between professional cultures as the social meaning of error shifts. Work in this context has been undertaken by one of the authors to show how medical professionals explain, rationalize, and normalize errors in their practice and how this relates to the maintenance of social status and identity (Waring 2004a). Ethnographic research provides an in-depth and contextualized approach for exploring the interpretation and the negotiation of meaning within particular social settings. This is particularly relevant for current patient safety research with its focus on organizational and professional cultures.

Cultures of collegiality and safety

How social meaning and values are shared within a social group is fundamental to their cultural make-up. The sharing of values and beliefs can be wide-ranging and can serve to reinforce collective social practice and define professional boundaries. For medicine, the concept of 'collegiality' is particularly significant in describing the collective sense of togetherness and belonging within the profession. Becker et al.'s (1961) ethnographic study of medical training shows how medical students *become* doctors not only through acquiring the necessary expertise and experience, but also through learning the collective beliefs, assumptions and symbolic rituals of the profession, including behaviour with patients, professional etiquette and conduct relating to the regulation of performance. As well as merely highlighting shared beliefs, the concept of collegiality and 'collegial culture' has come to describe how professional attitudes and practices serve to maintain the internalized and 'closed' control of occupational performance and exclude non-professional groups. For example, Arluke's (1977) ethnographic research illustrates how the collegial rituals of the surgical 'death round' functioned to normalize patient death and de-emphasize the relationship between death and professional conduct. These closed professional conferences represented a vehicle for professional learning and advancement through the identification of unusual physiology or technical complications: through the symbolic redefinition of poor performance as reasonable conduct under difficult circumstances. As such, the exclusionary collegial practices served to deflect and conceal unsafe and dangerous practice and in so doing, maintain professional authority and competence. Rosenthal (1995) has also investigated the way in which the medical profession deals with 'problem doctors'. Based on mainly interview data, she shows that the permanent uncertainty of medical knowledge and practice renders medicine inevitably error-prone. As such, medical culture has come to tolerate certain levels of wrong-doing, while reinforcing a norm of professional non-criticism. However, it is also shown how persistent issues of wrong-doing are typically addressed through 'in-house' collegial practices that serve to maintain the exclusivity of medical knowledge while simultaneously limiting exposure to non-professional groups.

The collegial culture of medicine is highly significant in the enhancement of healthcare quality and safety. The findings of the Bristol Royal Infirmary Inquiry suggest that the 'closed collegiality' of medicine, the assumption that 'doctor knows best' and a 'fear of blame' limit a more appropriate response to learning. Specifically the creation of a 'safety culture' is now a priority for health policy. However, it is first important to recognize the long-standing shared beliefs and practice that characterize the cultures of health care, in order to understand how they may diverge or resist current attempts to promote a new style of organizational learning. Within this context ethnographic research has further explored how recent developments in risk management are potentially limited by the shared beliefs and preference of doctors.

In addition to a 'fear of blame' doctors were discouraged from incident reporting because these systems were seen as non-medical and bureaucratic; lacking both the sense of purpose and confidentiality that characterized established collegial practices (Waring 2004a, 2005). More than necessarily a fear of blame, doctors were found to share an apprehension about managerial and bureaucratic systems that did not foster a shared culture, while more collegial forms of quality improvement were favoured because of a shared sense of purpose in collegial practices to make meaningful service improvements. Through both observations and interviews, ethnographic research can provide opportunities to explore how individuals come to acquire collective beliefs and conform to established social practices and rituals.

Teamwork and professional cultures

Teamwork is recognized as central to patient safety, and if we are to understand and change the nature of practice, we need to first examine the socio-cultural facets that underlie and shape this. Professional groups have sets of cultural norms originating in their distinct histories, training and roles which also provide for a set of relations between them that can facilitate or hinder teamwork. Hierarchical relations and rigid boundaries between healthcare professionals are a cultural barrier to effective teamwork, impacting upon sharing knowledge, decision-making, recognizing and learning from mistakes and communication. Moving beyond static snapshot measures of culture offered by surveys, ethnography can provide rich insights into the complexity of inter-professional work practices, relations and the meanings reflected and reproduced therein within specific contexts. In this section, we draw upon ethnographies conducted in the operating theatre and intensive care unit (ICU) to demonstrate the nature and value of this contribution to understandings of patient safety.

The importance of multi-disciplinary teamwork and knowledge sharing in the ICU has been emphasized. Utilizing participant observation, interviews and documentation to examine decision-making processes in ICU, Coombs and Ersser (2004) showed how doctors and nurses use different types of knowledge, and while pivotal, the nursing perspective is devalued. The dominance of the medical perspective reproduces boundaries between doctors and nurses, such that 'the reality of interdisciplinary working in ICU was not found to reflect the policy vision' (2004: 251), with 'fundamental ramifications for the quality of team decision making and effectiveness of new ways of professional working' (2004: 245). Melia (2001), however, used ethnographic interviews with ICU nurses to examine ethical decision-making and showed how doctor–nurse boundaries become blurred by virtue of all team members' efforts to avoid conflict and strive for moral consensus in the interests of good patient care. Ethical decisions are treated as a collective responsibility, which is a crucial means through which teamwork is preserved in the face of temporary disagreements and lapses in professional relations.

Ethnographies have also examined the socio-cultural aspects of inter-professional work in the operating theatre, highlighting ways in which 'subjectivities' of occupational groups are reflected and reproduced in everyday practices. In *The Social Meaning of Surgery*, Fox (1992) used ethnographic interviews and observations to examine the constitution of social relations in surgery as an inherently collaborative activity. He showed that professional groups hold different meanings or 'discourses' around work and the patient, but these manifest themselves in ways that serve to constitute the power and authority of surgery as a 'healing' speciality and downgrade its injuring nature, for example, in surgeon–anaesthetist interactions and theatre team hygiene practices. Finn (2003) examined cultural aspects of teamwork in the operating theatre using participant observation and found inherent conflict between occupational groups concerning the nature of work processes around the meaning of time, space and 'teamwork' itself. Conflict is managed so that it does not manifest itself openly, maintaining a definition of the group as a 'team' to enable cooperation. However, interests are pursued in more subverted ways that reflect and reproduce occupational boundaries and ultimately affect the efficiency and quality of teamwork, for example, through use of resources and knowledge sharing. Thus, while teamwork is valued, its effectiveness is undermined through the pursuit of diverse occupational objectives and specific issues in work processes.

Future challenges

Ethnography has a great deal to offer patient safety research. Unlike other research methods it offers an 'insider' perspective on the social world, almost enabling the researcher to 'get under the skin' of social actors and share in their cultural values, beliefs and practices. As shown above, this is primarily achieved through observing and participating in the social setting as it naturally occurs, to identify the social practices, rituals, routines and ceremonies that characterize social practice, and listening and talking both informally and formally with its members to understand how they make sense and give meaning to the world around them.

These socio-cultural dimensions are of central relevance to patient safety research. It is well established that the threats to patient safety are rarely the consequence of a single individual's behaviour but are the product of the complex individual, team-based, technical, managerial, organizational and institutional factors that characterize healthcare delivery (Department of Health 2000). A central object-ive of health service research is to understand how these multifaceted and multi-dimensional factors combine to threaten and also improve patient safety. It remains important to bear in mind, however, that culture, whether at the group, professional, or organizational levels, permeates all aspects of patient safety, whether it be how an individual perceives, interprets and makes sense of the threats to safety, the rituals and shared norms of teamwork, the priorities and value of management decision-making, the legitimacy of leadership and authority, the uptake and use of technological devices or the occupational response to organizational change. Ethnography therefore offers a rich, in-depth and holistic approach to studying health care and issues of patient safety as it naturally occurs, investigating and making explicit the shared assumptions, beliefs and values that emerge through and inform everyday social practice. In this sense it promises to reach parts of the social world other methods cannot reach.

The centrality of culture to patient safety is further demonstrated by its import-ance in health policy. Not only have policies highlighted the significant of a 'blame culture' in inhibiting the improvement of safety, but it recommends the creation of a 'safety culture' whereby healthcare professionals share in the values of openness, reporting and learning, thereby facilitating the introduction of incident reporting and proactive risk management systems. Again, ethnography has much to offer patient safety research in this area, exploring the extent to which it is feasible to foster these values within the health service, to explore the barriers and facilitators to change and to determine what impact new patient safety systems are having on healthcare cultures.

Although our argument is that ethnography can make a unique contribution to the study of culture, and therefore the patient safety agenda, this does not mean that it cannot be used in conjunction with other methods. Indeed, value can be gained through the complementary use of ethnography alongside other methods within any research project, for example, to give greater depth and understanding of issues highlighted by survey or structured interview data (e.g. safety 'climate') or to provide a basis from which those instruments can be designed in an informed way. This is not a simple task of triangulation to achieve one set of findings, but rather to provide a richer and broader insight into the social world by revealing those aspects not captured by other methods.

Ethnography is not without its challenges. It is not a quick and easy approach, but can be demanding on time, resources and the individual researcher in the field. It requires a level of skill and understanding of the approach among those conducting the research, and an ability to deal with the ongoing practical, ethical and theoretical issues that arise during the course of study. Furthermore, in using ethnography to inform policy, the issue of generalizability of substantive findings from in-depth case studies to wider settings becomes a pertinent one, and requires informed judge-ment regarding sampling and as to those aspects of the field and social group researched that are relevant and similar to other settings (Hammersley 1992). However, the rewards offered by ethnography are great and it offers insights into the socio-cultural worlds of healthcare organizations potentially not possible through other methodologies.

Box 12.1 Key points

- Ethnography is particularly suited to exploring the in-depth and contextualized aspects of healthcare cultures as they naturally occur, including the values, beliefs, meanings that make up social cultures and relate to patient safety.
- Ethnography involves acquiring a detailed and 'insider's' perspective on the social world, through the use of observations, interviews and the collection of cultural artefacts.
- Ethnographic analysis is ongoing and iterative alongside data collection. It is inductive, with its concepts emergent, grounded and developed in data.
- Ethnographic research has shown how the perception and interpretation of the threats to patient safety are informed by their wider socio-cultural context.
- Ethnographic research explores the social norms, rules and rituals related to the management of healthcare safety.
- Ethnography can show how teamwork practices emerge from multiple professional cultures and their negotiation in everyday practice.
- Ethnography's in-depth nature makes demands on researcher time, resources and skills.
- Ethnography's in-depth and holistic approach can add greater cultural understanding to other tools and measures of patient safety.

References

Arluke, A. (1977) Social control rituals in medicine: the case of the surgical death rounds, in R. Dingwall, C. Heath, M. Reid and M. Stacey (eds) *Health Care and Health Knowledge*. London: Croom Helm.

Becker, H., Geer, B., Hughes, E. and Strauss, A. (1961) *Boys in White: Student Culture in Medical School*. Chicago: University of Chicago Press.

Berger, P. and Luckman, T. (1967) *The Social Construction of Reality*. Harmondsworth: Penguin.

Bosk, C. (1979) *Forgive and Remember*. London: University of Chicago Press.

Bosk, C. (1986) Professional responsibility and medical error, in L. Aiken and D. Mechanic (eds) *Applications of Social Science to Clinical Medicine and Health Policy*. New Brunswisk, NJ: Rutgers University Press.

Brewer, J.D. (2000) *Ethnography*. Buckingham: Open University Press.

Burgess, R.G. (1984) *In the Field: An Introduction to Field Research*. London: Unwin Hyman.

Coombs, M. and Ersser, S.J. (2004) Medical hegemony in decision making – a barrier to interdisciplinary working in intensive care? *Journal of Advanced Nursing*, 46(3): 245–52.

Department of Health (2000) *An Organization with a Memory*. London: The Stationery Office.

Dingwall, R. and Finn, R. (2000) Organizational culture. http://www.bristol-inquiry.org.uk/seminars/brisph2_seminar3points.htm

Fetterman, D. (1989) *Ethnography: Step by Step*. London: Sage.

Finn, R. (2003) Collaborative work in the operating theatre: conflict and the discourse of teamwork, unpublished PhD thesis, Nottingham University.

Fox, N. (1992) *The Social Meaning of Surgery*. Buckingham: Open University Press.

Fox, R. (2000) Medical uncertainty revisited, in G. Albrecht and R. Fitzpatrick (eds) *A Sociology of Medical Practice*. London: Collier-Macmillan.

Freidson, E. (1975) *Doctoring Together: A Study of Professional Social Control*. New York: Elsevier.

Geertz, C. (1973) *The Interpretation of Cultures*. New York: Basic Books.

Glaser, B.G. and Strauss, A.L. (1967) *The Discovery of Grounded Theory*. Chicago: Aldine.

Gold, R. (1969) Roles in sociological field observations, in G. McCall (ed.) *Issues in Participant Observations*. London: Addison-Wesley.

Hammersley, M. (1992) *What's Wrong with Ethnography?* London: Routledge.

Hammersley, M. and Atkinson, P. (1995) *Ethnography: Principles in Practice*. 2nd edn. London: Routledge.

Helmreich, R. and Merritt, A. (1998) *Culture at Work in Aviation and Medicine*. Aldershot: Ashgate.

Melia, K.M. (2001) Ethical issues and the importance of consensus in the intensive care team, *Social Science and Medicine*, 53: 707–19.

National Patient Safety Agency (2003) *Seven Steps to Patient Safety*. London: NPSA.

Paget, M. (2004) *The Unity of Mistakes*. Philadelphia, PA: Temple University Press.

Reason, J. (1997) *Managing the Risks of Organizational Accidents*. Aldershot: Ashgate.

Rosenthal, M. (1995) *The Incompetent Doctor*. Buckingham: Open University Press.

Schatzman, L. and Strauss, A. (1973) *Field Research: Strategies for Natural Sociology*. Englewood Cliffs, NJ: Prentice-Hall.

Silverman, D. (1993) *Interpreting Qualitative Data: Methods for Analysing Talk, Text and Interaction*. London: Sage.

Waring, J. (2004a) The Social Construction and Control of Medical Errors: a new frontier for medical/managerial relations, unpublished thesis, University of Nottingham.

Waring, J. (2004b) A qualitative study of the intra-hospital variations in incident reporting, *International Journal of Quality in Health Care*, 16(5): 347–52.

Waring, J. (2005) Beyond blame: the cultural barriers to medical incident reporting, *Social Science and Medicine*, 60(9): 1927–35.

13

Evaluating safety culture

Susan Kirk, Martin Marshall, Tanya Claridge, Aneez Esmail and Dianne Parker

Until recently, those working in patient safety have largely focussed on the more mechanistic aspects of the field, such as the epidemiology of adverse events and the introduction of technical innovations aimed at preventing these events. However, we are now seeing an increasing emphasis being placed on the importance of understanding the shared attitudes, beliefs, values and assumptions that underlie how people perceive and act upon safety issues within their organizations and on the potential importance of these shared characteristics to initiating fundamental and sustained changes to patient safety (Department of Health 2000; Leape and Berwick 2000; Vincent et al. 2000). These shared characteristics are referred to as the 'safety culture' of an organization (Pidgeon 1991; Clarke 1999; Mearns et al. 2003).

Organizational safety culture: concept and characteristics

Interest in organizational culture has a long history in disciplines such as sociology and organizational studies, for example, in the work of Hofstede (1980) and Schein (1985). There is now increasing interest in applying and extending this work to the health sector (Scott et al. 2003a; Mannion et al. 2004). Many of the issues that have been explored in other fields, are now being revisited by health service researchers. Most fundamentally, the concept of an organization having a 'culture' is contested and there is an on-going polarized debate between those who see culture as a variable that can be manipulated and measured ('what an organization has') and those who see it as a descriptive metaphor ('what an organization is') (Davies et al. 2000). Despite this philosophical tension, there is a common agreement that culture can be conceptualized as the shared beliefs, norms and values of the people who work in an organization and it is generally accepted that organizational culture has the potential to influence their actions and patterns of communication (Leape and Berwick 2000; Wilson 2001; Clarke 2003; Scott et al. 2003a).

In organizations where operations may involve risk for staff or the public, it is helpful to consider that there is an organizational culture specifically related to safety – a 'safety culture' (Moran and Volkwein 1992; Leape and Berwick 2000; Hart and Hazelgrove 2001; Clarke 2003; Nieva and Sorra 2003). It is thus one element of the broader construct of organizational culture. The safety culture of an organization is expressed through a range of interrelated aspects, some of which are organization specific, and some of which are generic; some aspects relate to the behaviour of members of the organization and some relate to the systems and processes in place to manage safety. These aspects include communication; perceptions of the importance of safety; confidence in the efficacy of preventative (safety) measures; organizational learning; leadership and executive responsibility; and the approach to incident reporting and analysis (Leape and Berwick 2000; Carroll et al. 2002; Kuhn and Youngberg 2002; Singer et al. 2003). Developments and changes in practices and procedures within the organization are thought to both shape and reflect the safety culture in a dynamic and evolving way. In complex organizations there are both tangible aspects of safety culture (for example, how incidents are investigated), and more abstract ones (for example, the priority given to safety).

The viability of developing a positive safety culture is thought to be influenced by the quality of staff–management communications, agreement at all levels of the organization that safety is important and confidence that safety measures are adequate (Caroll et al. 2002; Kuhn and Youngberg 2002). The characteristics of an organization with a positive safety culture are described in Box 13.1 (Health and Safety Commission 1993; Leape and Berwick 2000; Carol et al. 2002; Kuhn and Youngberg 2002; Nieva and Sorra 2003; Singer et al. 2003; Westrum 2004). Given the complexity and multi-dimensionality of safety culture, it is perhaps not surprising that there is little guidance or useful models available to organizations and front-line staff on how to improve their safety culture (Clarke 1999; Hale 2000).

Box 13.1 Characteristics of a positive safety culture

- Communication founded on mutual trust and openness
- Good information flow and processing
- Shared perceptions of the importance of safety
- Recognition of the inevitability of error
- Confidence in the efficacy of preventative (safety) measures
- Proactive identification of latent threats to safety
- Organizational learning
- Committed leadership and executive responsibility
- A 'no blame', non-punitive approach to incident reporting and analysis.

The importance of safety culture

Safety culture is an interesting concept, but is it an important one in terms of the management of risk in healthcare organizations? Experts in risk management, both inside and outside health care, have emphasized the importance of considering system failures and system-driven errors over direct human error, and they have highlighted the crucial role that organizational culture plays in ensuring that the system is safe (Clarke 2003). As a result, safety culture is generally seen as being fundamental to the ability of an organization to manage the safety of its operations (Cox and Flin

1998; Cox and Cheyne 2000; Glendon and Stanton 2000). As a result, a great deal of effort has been expended on initiatives aimed at improving the safety culture of health organizations. These have included incident and error-reporting mechanisms, development of root cause analysis tools, and encouraging active learning following adverse events and near misses (Brennan et al. 1991; Bhasale et al. 1998; Mustard 2002; Ruffles 2002; Bird and Milligan 2003). However, the extent to which there is a cultural dimension to these initiatives is unclear.

There is some research evidence to suggest that developing a positive safety culture may help to improve safety performance, although demonstrating a causal link has proved problematic (Seppälä 1997; Griffin and Neal 2000; Sorenson 2002). Looking at the broader concept of organizational culture, a recent review of empirical studies exploring the relationship between organizational culture and performance concluded that the relationship is not strong, is complex and is contingent on the specific kind of culture and performance being investigated (Scott et al. 2003b). Even the face validity of using culture as a lever for improvement is unclear. For example, in a study examining the importance of culture to primary care managers in the United Kingdom, Marshall and colleagues found that managers saw culture as an important concept but not one that could be manipulated in any predictable way (Marshall et al. 2002). Assuming that these findings are applicable to the specific field of safety culture, it seems unlikely that there is a simple or direct relationship between a safe culture and safe practice in healthcare organizations.

Approaches to evaluating safety cultures in health care

A large number of tools with differing characteristics have been developed to assess the generic concept of organizational culture (Scott et al. 2003a). However, none of these instruments make explicit reference to safety culture. It is only in recent years that instruments have started to be developed to specifically measure the safety culture of healthcare organizations (Spurgeon et al. 1999; Nieva 2002; Gaba et al. 2003; Nieva and Sorra 2003; Singer et al. 2003; Sorra and Nieva 2004; Weingart et al. 2004). In this chapter we will describe three different safety culture assessment tools, identifying their similarities, differences and applications. These tools have been selected because they are illustrative of the range of instruments currently available. For example, one is an established tool while the other tools are new; one is a typographical tool and the other are dimensional; two tools have an explicit theoretical basis; one tool aims to help staff understand and reflect on safety culture and promote discussion about ways of improving it within their teams or organizations.

The Hospital Survey on Patient Safety Culture (HSPSC)

The HSPSC has recently been developed by American researchers (Sorra and Nieva 2004) and funded by the Agency for Healthcare Quality and Research (AHRQ). It aims to enable organizations to assess their own safety culture (and track changes in this over time) and evaluate the impact of patient safety interventions. It has no explicit theoretical framework and was developed from a review of the literature and existing safety culture surveys followed by interviews with hospital staff. The resulting survey instrument was then pretested and piloted and the data analysed using factor analyses to identify which items and scales to retain.

The tool contains 44 items reflecting a comprehensive range of safety culture dimensions (Table 13.1). Respondents rate their agreement to the statements on a 5-point Likert scale and frequencies can be produced for each dimension. It is designed for use by a range of staff at different levels within an organization. The tool enables team and organizational culture to be examined and the analysis of differences between teams and between teams and the wider organizational culture.

It has been designed for use in the acute sector and its terminology reflects this aim. As it is a new tool, there is a lack of information on its practical uses or on perceptions of its appropriateness. The tool and a detailed guide to how it can be used is available without charge from the AHRQ website (http://www.ahcpr.gov/qual/hospculture/).

The Safety Climate Survey (SCS)

The SCS was developed by Sexton et al. (2000, 2003) at the University of Texas Center of Excellence for Patient Safety Research and Practice. It aims to allow organizations to be able to assess staff perceptions of safety culture and to monitor the success of the introduction of patient safety initiatives.

It is derived from the Flight Management and Attitudes Safety Survey (FMASS) (Sexton et al. 2001), a widely used and well recognized aviation tool that examines cockpit management attitudes. The FMASS was developed to measure attitudes to status hierarchies, leadership, interpersonal interaction and attitudes to stress. It has been reported that this tool has good test–retest reliability and internal consistency and that it is predictive of performance and accident rates (Sexton et al. 2000;

Table 13.1 A comparison of the patient safety culture dimensions assessed by the tools

Patient safety dimensions/components	Tools		
	HSPCS	SCS	MaPSaF
Communication	✔	✔	✔
Priority given to patient safety	✔	✔	✔
Perception of the causes of patient safety incidents	✔	✔	✔
Personnel management	✔		✔
Leadership	✔	✔	✔
Training and education			✔
Learning from patient safety incidents		✔	✔
Physical work environment	✔		
Teamwork	✔		✔
Identification of the causes of patient safety incidents			✔
Incident reporting	✔	✔	✔
Information processing	✔		✔
Patient involvement			✔
Error management	✔	✔	✔

Pronovost et al. 2003). Many of the safety culture tools that have been developed are similarly theoretically underpinned by aviation research or research relating to high-risk industries.

The SCS contains contains 19 items relating to safety culture dimensions and respondents rate their agreement to these statements on a 5-point Likert scale. Scores can then be aggregated to produce an overall safety culture score. The tool allows for differences in safety culture to be investigated between teams and the wider organization. The developers recommend that a baseline measurement is collected followed by six monthly or annual surveys to assess the impact of initiatives. Like the HSPSC, the tool has been designed for use in the acute hospital setting although the terminology is reasonably generic. It appears to be less comprehensive in terms of the dimensions of safety culture than the other two tools described in this chapter.

The SCS has been used in research and in clinical settings across the United States of America and in Europe (for example, Pronovost et al. 2003). It is available from the Institute of Healthcare Improvement's website following registration with the site along with guides to its implementation and analysis (http://www.ihi.org/IHI/Topics/PatientSafety/).

Manchester Patient Safety Assessment Framework (MaPSaF)

MaPSaF has been developed by the authors of this chapter at the National Primary Care Research and Development Centre, University of Manchester. This tool aims to help front-line clinicians and managers engage with the concept of safety culture and enable them to qualitatively assess and reflect on the patient safety culture within their team or organization and consider how it can be improved. Apart from the Strategies for Leadership Scale (SLS) (VHA/AHA 2000), it appears to be the only tool that provides a 'road map' of how an organization can improve its safety culture and how an 'ideal' organization might be portrayed. It is the only tool which has an explicit aim of 'unpacking' the concept of safety culture in order to make it more accessible to clinicians and managers.

Originally the tool was developed for use in UK primary care sector. This was because it was recognized that the potential for safety problems in primary care is significant, not just because of the volume of patient contacts but also because of the complexity of primary care and the level of uncertainty associated with providing care in a community setting. Moreover, the concept of an organization in UK primary care is particularly complex and is not a discrete, easily defined or measured unit. Networked organizations called Primary Care Trusts (PCTs) are responsible for the management of groups of general practices, community nursing services, pharmacies and other diverse community health services in a defined geographical area. Healthcare professionals operate within and between multiple practices and teams and undertake both routine care and increasingly 'high-tech' activities on a day-to-day basis. Different cultural influences operate across and within professional groups, within and between practices and teams, and between the front-line services and the PCT management, resulting in the existence of multiple micro-cultures. In addition, the majority of safety culture assessment tools have been developed for use in the US healthcare system and we felt that it was important to develop a tool that was grounded in the reality of clinicians and managers who were working in the UK National Health Service.

The theory underpinning the tool was originally developed by Westrum (1993) and later adapted by Parker and Hudson (2001). Westrum proposed that one way of distinguishing between organizational cultures is to examine the ways in which information is handled by the organization and he identified three different cultures which he called pathological, bureaucratic and generative. He regarded the ways in which information is processed within organizations as fundamental because of its close association with other features of an organization's culture (Westrum 2004). Parker and Hudson's empirical work in the petro-chemical industry extended this framework to five levels (Table 13.2) and applied their new framework more generally to the safety culture of organizations. They proposed a model in which a range of safety activities might be characterized at five levels of organizational safety culture maturity. For each of these activities, the organization will be at one of the five levels of safety culture maturity. Such a typology is useful in understanding organizational safety culture (Westrum 2004) and we thought that it was potentially applicable to our work.

The nine dimensions describing safety culture in primary care organizations were developed from a comprehensive review of the literature and from consultation with national opinion leaders in patient safety. These dimensions then formed the framework for qualitative semi-structured interviews conducted with a purposeful sample of managers and clinicians from different professional groups working within PCTs and local practices. The interviews drew upon participants' experience and expertise in order to develop descriptions of what an organization might look like for each of the nine dimensions at each of the five levels of organizational maturity. In addition, the face validity of the dimensions were further explored. The final tool is presented in the form of a Guttman-type matrix with the five levels of maturity as one axis and the nine dimensions of patient safety as the other.

While the tool was originally developed for use in primary care, further versions have now been developed for use in acute care, mental health services and ambulance services. Further work has also been conducted to establish the face and content

Table 13.2 Levels of organizational safety culture

Level of organizational safety culture	Characterization
LEVEL 1: Pathological	Why do we need to waste our time on risk management and safety issues?
LEVEL 2: Reactive	We take risk seriously and do something every time we have an incident.
LEVEL 3: Calculative	We have systems in place to manage all likely risks.
LEVEL 4: Proactive	We are always on the alert, thinking of risks that might emerge.
LEVEL 5: Generative	Risk management is an integral part of everything we do.

Source: Parker and Hudson (2001)

validity of the tool. We are currently planning a quantitative evaluation in order to examine the coherence and internal consistency of the statements making up each descriptor and the relationship between the different levels of maturity. This may then result in the development of a new quantitative instrument, derived from and related to the qualitative framework.

We plan to provide a downloadable copy of the tool on the Internet and to produce a guide to its application. MaPSaF has not been used as a research instrument but it will be used by the National Patient Safety Agency (NPSA) across the NHS from 2005. Table 13.3 summarizes the differences and similarities between the three tools.

Future challenges

To date, only a small number of tools have been developed to assess the safety culture of healthcare organizations and workgroups. They all have limitations in their scope, ease of use or in terms of the investigation of their scientific properties. Which tool to use largely depends on the purpose of the study or assessment, its methodological approach and the resources available (Nieva and Sorra 2003; Scott et al. 2003a). Some researchers may wish to develop and use a numerical scoring tool while others may prefer a more qualitative approach, rejecting the idea that it is possible to measure a complex phenomenon such as safety culture (Scott et al. 2003a).

Most tools consist of two types of statements representing safety culture dimensions – statements relating to values, beliefs and attitudes and statements relating to actual safety behaviours that aim to improve safety (for example, structures, policies). While the number of items vary, the dimensions are fairly consistent across the tools and many appear to be transferable between different types of teams, organizations, care sectors and countries. However, there are differences in how comprehensively they cover these dimensions with MaPSaF being particularly comprehensive. Another tool not reviewed in this chapter, the SLS, covers all the dimensions identified in Table 13.1 and, like MaPSaF, enables identification of the actions needed to improve safety culture. However, it is possibly less transferable as it uses North American-specific terminology.

There are also differences in the fundamental approach taken to assessing safety culture. MaPSaF takes a typological approach in that assessment results in one or more 'types' of cultures. Other tools such as the SCS and the HSPCS take a dimensional approach, with safety culture being described in terms of its position on a number of continuous variables. Indeed, the vast majority of safety culture assessment tools are designed in the form of survey questionnaires and focus on assessing the opinions of individual members of staff to a series of predetermined statements about safety and result in a numerical score that is said to indicate the strength of the safety culture present in the organization. The responses therefore represent a snapshot of individuals' current perceptions of the superficial manifestations of safety culture (the so-called 'safety climate'), emphasizing individual attitudes and opinions, rather than their shared beliefs, values and assumptions. They therefore fail to evaluate the deeper – and probably more important – manifestations of the culture of an organization. They also fail to take account of the complexity of interactions between staff members

Table 13.3 Similarities and differences between the three tools

Characteristic	HSPSC	SCS	MaPSaF
Country of origin	USA	USA	UK
Purpose	Safety culture assessment and evaluation of the impact of interventions (including longitudinal assessment)	Assessment of staff perceptions of safety culture and monitoring the success of the introduction of patient safety initiatives	Qualitative assessment and self-reflection of patient safety culture and how improvements can be made
Theoretical framework	None explicit	Aviation research Developed from the FMASS	Westrum's organizational maturity continuum
Nature	Dimensional Quantitative	Dimensional Quantitative	Typological Qualitative
Format	44 item self-completion questionnaire using a 5-point Likert scale	19 item self-completion questionnaire using a 5-point Likert scale	9 × 5 matrix with safety culture dimensions on one axis and different levels of safety culture maturity on the other
Level of analysis	At both the team level and the wider organization	At both the team level and the wider organization (by using ANOVA based on demographic data)	Explicitly designed to enable analysis at level of team, location or wider organization
Scientific properties	Reliability of dimensions .63–.84 (Crohnbach's alpha). Cognitive testing ('Think aloud'). Construct validity	FMASS has good test–retest reliability and internal consistency. Predictive of performance and accident rates	Face and content validity established. Criterion validity to be explored
Healthcare application	Acute sector	Acute sector	Primary care originally but versions now developed for acute sector, mental health services and ambulance service

within organizations, the differing influence of individuals and professional groups on culture and the emergent nature of safety culture.

Tools also vary in the extent to which they are designed to assess the safety culture of subgroups within an organization, whether they have a strong theoretical and conceptual background and the extent to which their validity and reliability have been evaluated (Table 13.3). Most of the currently available instruments have been designed in the USA for use in acute hospitals and may not be generalizable to other countries and to non-hospital organizations such as those delivering primary care services.

More research is required to produce valid and reliable tools that can be used in a wide range of contexts and which could be used to evaluate the impact of a range of interventions to improve safety culture. However, it is our contention that in order to develop an understanding of the subtleties and multi-dimensional nature of safety culture in healthcare organizations, a more sophisticated approach is needed than the use of self-report questionnaires alone (Marshall et al. 2003). As Scott et al. (2003a) note, a multi-method approach will always be desirable in order to obtain a valid, reliable and trustworthy assessment of such a nebulous concept. Triangulating between different methods is the best way of understanding a complex phenomenon. Qualitative methods such as interviewing and documentary analysis allow researchers to obtain a deeper understanding about how staff construct the safety culture within their team or organization, while observation enables them to examine what actually happens. It is the congruents and discongruents between these different methods that give us insight. Consequently, if we are to obtain a holistic understanding of safety culture within teams and organizations, or if we are attempting to improve patient safety, safety culture assessment instruments should form only one part of our toolkit.

Box 13.2 Key points

- Organizational culture has been studied by a number of disciplines over many years and is generally conceptualized as the shared beliefs, norms and values of the people who work in an organization.
- One element of organizational culture is safety culture, expressed through a range of interrelated aspects – the behaviours, beliefs and values of members of the organization regarding safety and the systems and processes in place to manage safety.
- Developing an effective safety culture is important to making lasting improvements in patient safety.
- A small number of tools have been developed in an attempt to assess and measure organizational safety culture, mainly in the format of survey questionnaires that use Likert scales.
- Such tools are generally comprehensive and similar in the safety dimensions they cover but limited testing of the reliability and validity of tools has been conducted to date.
- Tools vary in terms of their theoretical underpinnings, the extent to which it is possible to assess micro cultures within organizations and their transferability within healthcare settings and systems.
- Which tool to use will depend on the purpose of the study or assessment, its methodological approach and the resources available.
- The nebulous, multi-dimensional nature of safety culture means that safety culture assessment instruments should form only one part of a multi-method toolkit to assess and improve patient safety.

References

Bhasale, A.L., Miller, G.C., Reid, S.E. and Britt, H.C. (1998) Analysing potential harm in Australian general practice: an incident monitoring study, *Medical Journal of Australia*, 169: 73–6.

Bird, D. and Milligan, F. (2003) Adverse health-care events: part 3. Learning the lessons, *Professional Nurse*, 18(11): 621–5.

Brennan, T.A., Leape, L.L., Laird, N.M., Hebert, L. and Localio, A.R. (1991) Incidence of adverse events and negligence in hospitalised patients: results of the Harvard medical practice study I, *New England Journal of Medicine*, 324: 377–84.

Caroll, J.S., Rudolph, J.W. and Hatakenaka, S. (2002) Lessons learned from non-medical industries: root cause analysis as cultural change at a chemical plant, *Quality and Safety in Health Care*, 11: 266–9.

Clarke, S. (1999) Perceptions of organizational safety: implications for the development of safety culture, *Journal of Organizational Behaviour*, 20: 185–98.

Clarke, S. (2003) The contemporary workforce: implications for organizational safety culture, *Personnel Review*, 32(1): 40–57.

Cox, S.J. and Cheyne, A.J.T. (2000) Assessing safety culture in offshore environments, *Safety Science*, 34: 111–29.

Cox, S.J. and Flin, R. (1998) Safety culture: philosopher's stone or man of straw? *Work and Stress*, 12(3): 189–201.

Davies, H.T.O., Nutley, S.M. and Mannion, R. (2000) Organizational culture and quality of health care, *Quality in Health Care*, 9: 111–19.

Department of Health (2000) *An Organization with a Memory: Report of an Expert Group on Learning from Adverse Events in the NHS*. London: The Stationery Office.

Gaba, D.M., Singer, S.J., Sinaiko, A.D., Bowen, J.D. and Ciavarelli, A.P. (2003) Differences in safety climate between hospital personnel and naval aviators, *Human Factors*, 45(2): 173–85.

Glendon, A.I. and Stanton, N.A. (2000) Perspectives on safety culture, *Safety Science*, 34: 193–214.

Griffin, M.A. and Neal, A. (2000) Perceptions of safety at work: a framework for linking safety climate to safety performance, knowledge, and motivation, *Journal of Occupational Health Psychology*, 5(3): 347–58.

Hale, A.R. (2000) Culture's confusions, *Safety Science*, 34: 1–14.

Hart, E. and Hazelgrove, J. (2001) Understanding the organizational context for adverse events in the health services: the role of cultural censorship, *Quality in Health Care*, 10: 257–62.

Health and Safety Commission (1993) *Organising for Safety: Third Report of the Human Factors Study Group of ACSNI*. Sudbury: HSE Books.

Hofstede, G. (1980) Values and culture, in G. Hofstede (ed.) *Culture's Consequences: International Differences in Work-Related Values*. Beverly Hills, CA: Sage, pp. 13–53.

Kuhn, A.M. and Youngberg, B.J. (2002) The need for risk management to evolve to assure a culture of safety, *Quality and Safety in Healthcare*, 11: 158–62.

Leape, L.L. and Berwick, D.M. (2000) Safe health care: are we up to it? *British Medical Journal*, 320: 725–6.

Mannion, R., Davies, H.T.O. and Marshall, M.N. (2004) *Cultures for Performance in Health Care*. Maidenhead: Open University Press.

Marshall, M., Sheaff, R., Rogers, A., Campbell, S., Halliwell, S., Pickard, S., Sibbald, B. and Roland, M. (2002) A qualitative study of the cultural changes in primary care organizations needed to implement clinical governance, *British Journal of General Practice*, 52(481): 641–5.

Marshall, M.N., Parker, D., Esmail, A., Kirk, S. and Claridge, T. (2003) Culture of safety, *Quality and Safety in Health Care*, 12: 318.

Mearns, K., Whittaker, S. and Flinn, R. (2003) Safety climate, safety management practice and safety performance in off shore environments, *Safety Science*, 41(8): 641–80.

Moran, E.T. and Volkwein, J.F. (1992) The cultural approach to the formation of organizational climate, *Human Relations*, 45(1): 19–46.

Mustard, L.W. (2002) The culture of patient safety, *JONA's Healthcare Law, Ethics, and Regulation*, 4(4): 111–15.

Nieva, V. (2002) *United States/United Kingdom Patient Safety Research Methodology Workshop: Measuring Patient Safety Culture*. Rockville, MD: The Agency for Healthcare Research and Quality/The Patient Safety Research Programme.

Nieva, V.F. and Sorra, J. (2003) Safety culture assessment: a tool for improving patient safety culture in healthcare organizations, *Quality and Safety in Health Care*, 12(Suppl II): 17–23.

Parker, D. and Hudson, P.T. (2001) *HSE: Understanding your Culture*. Rijswijk, the Netherlands: Shell International Exploration and Production, EP 2001–5124.

Pidgeon, N.F. (1991) Safety culture and risk management in organizations, *Journal of Cross-Cultural Psychology*, 22(1): 129–40.

Provonost, P.J., Weast, B., Holzmueller, C.G., Rosenstein, B.J., Kidwell, R.P., Haller, K.B., Feroli, E.R., Sexton, J.B. and Rubin, H.R. (2003) Evaluation of the culture of safety: survey of clinicians and managers in an academic medical center, *Quality and Safety in Health Care*, 12: 405–10.

Ruffles, S. (2002) Promoting patient safety in primary care: Practices should set up their own critical incident reporting (Letter), *British Medical Journal*, 324(7329): 109.

Schein, E. (1985) *Organizational Culture and Leadership*. San Francisco: Jossey-Bass.

Scott, T., Mannion, R., Davies, H. and Marshall, M. (2003a) The quantitative measurement of organizational culture in health care: a review of the available instruments, *Health Services Researcher*, 38: 923–45.

Scott, T., Mannion, R., Marshall, M. and Davies, H. (2003b) Does organizational culture influence health care performance? A review of the evidence, *Journal of Health Services and Research Policy*, 8(2): 105–17.

Seppälä, A. (1997) Safety management and accident prevention: safety culture in 14 small and medium-sized companies, in P. Seppälä, T. Luopajarvi, C.H. Nygard and M. Mattila (eds) *From Experience to Innovation, IEA '97, Vol. 3* (pp. 285–7). Helsinki: Finnish Institute of Occupational Health.

Sexton, J.B., Helmreich, R. and Williams, R. (2001) *The Flight Management Attitudes Safety Survey (FMASS)*. Austin, TXs: University of Texas Press.

Sexton, J.B., Thomas, E.J. and Helmreich, R. (2000) Error, stress and teamwork in medicine and aviation: cross-sectional surveys, *British Medical Journal*, 320: 745–9.

Sexton, J.B. and Thomas, E.J. (2003) *The Safety Climate Survey: Psychometric and Benchmarking Properties*. Austin, TX: The University of Texas Center of Excellence for Patient Safety Research and Practice.

Singer, S.J., Gaba, D.M., Geppert, J.J., Sinaiko, A.D., Howard, S.K. and Park, K.C. (2003) The culture of safety: results of an organization-wide survey in 15 California hospitals. *Quality and Safety in Health Care*, 12(2): 112–18.

Sorenson, J.N. (2002) Safety culture: a survey of the state-of-the-art. *Reliable Engineering System Safety*, 76: 189–204.

Sorra, J. and Nieva, V. (2004) *Hospital Survey on Patient Safety Culture*. Rockville, MD: Agency for Healthcare Research and Quality.

Spurgeon, P., Barwell, F., Parker, L. and Dineen, M. (1999) *Organizational Culture and its Potential Relationship to Clinical Risk*. Birmingham: Health Services Management Centre: University of Birmingham.

VHA/American Hospital Association (AHA) (2000) *Strategies for Leadership: An Organizational Approach to Patient Safety*. Chicago: American Hospital Association.

Vincent, C., Taylor-Adams, S., Chapman, E.J., Hewett, D., Prior, S., Strange, P. and Tizzard, A. (2000) How to investigate and analyse clinical incidents: clinical risk management unit and association of litigation and risk management protocol, *British Medical Journal*, 320: 777–81.

Weingart, S.N., Farbstein, K., Davis, R.B. and Phillips, R.S. (2004) Using a multihospital survey to examine the safety culture, *Joint Commission Journal on Quality and Safety*, 30: 125–32.

Westrum, R. (1993) Cultures with requisite imagination, in J.A. Wise, V.D. Hopkin and P. Stager (eds) *Verification and Validation of Complex Systems: Human Factors Issues* (pp. 401–16). Berlin: Springer-Verlag.

Westrum, R. (2004) A typology of organizational cultures, *Quality and Safety in Health Care*, 13(Suppl. II): 22–7.

Wilson, A.M. (2001) Understanding organizational culture and the implications for corporate marketing, *European Journal of Marketing*, 35(3–4): 353–67.

PART 3
Patient safety in practice

14

Patient safety
Education, training and professional development

Amanda Howe

> We certify practitioners as ready to provide high-quality care. Yet we have not done much in those training programs to systematically review the causes of error; nor have we yet really developed methods for carefully identifying the factors that lead to error. Today there is little education about medical injury prevention in medical schools or training programs, and few signs of new efforts to do so. We need to change this by restructuring medical education to allow time for instruction in and discussion of quality issues and methods for improvement. Addressing medical errors is a compelling subject for such instruction. (Brennan 2002)

Threats to patient safety may arise from organizational errors, but organizations are made up of individuals, and it is individual attitudes and actions which contribute to error. Poor professional performance inevitably leads to questions about the training which clinical staff receive in patient safety issues – both in terms of its efficacy at preventing error, and as a solution to current problems. This chapter therefore addresses the role which formal undergraduate and postgraduate training plays in developing professional understanding of patient safety, and makes recommendations for curricular approaches and relevant educational methods to underpin both theoretical content and learning from clinical experience. It draws largely on examples from the clinical discipline of medicine, though many points will be generalizable to other health professionals.

Using education as a means of patient safety – rationale and assumptions

There are two main routes by which education contributes to patient safety: in the years of formal pre- and postgraduate training: and in experiential learning, including continuing professional development (CPD). The first approach assumes that formal training will develop habitual responses that can help to protect patients from risk over a lifetime of practice. The consequence of this belief is to include patient safety as part of a formal curriculum (specific learning opportunities designed to highlight key concepts and relevant knowledge and skills).

Patient safety and the formal curriculum

Most training courses show very few taught components with titles such as 'patient safety', 'clinical error', or 'dealing with adverse events'. This is because large parts of clinical training are organized either around basic science themes (anatomy, physiology), body systems (cardiovascular, renal), the target patient group (child health, intensive care), or core specialty competencies (emergency caesarean section, cardiac catheterization). Modern curricula have become more problem focused and integrated, and learning is often built around patient problems (blackouts, chest pain). In such applied settings, a common response to the promotion of patient safety as a specific curricular theme is that 'everything we do is about patient safety already'. Hand washing, consultation skills, management of infusion devices, and potential drug interactions are all examples where poor knowledge and skills *could* result in an adverse event for a patient, and there can be very few content areas which could be dismissed on the grounds that they have no possible links with patient safety.

In principle, integrated approaches are entirely compatible with the demonstration of patient safety issues, but may feel risky to those who wish to make patient safety highly visible as a key theme in their curriculum. Also, over-inclusive generalizations do not help curriculum developers to decide whether the learning experiences offered to their students are adequately focused on safety issues, and whether the learners themselves can recognize and manage risk. It is therefore recommended that some part of a formal curriculum is explicitly focused on patient safety. The main arguments for a formal component on patient safety in any clinical training is that it makes the subject 'visible' to learners, and ensures that it appears in the formal learning outcomes – which means it will also be formally assessed. Novice learners often benefit from some didactic input on core topics and definitions in order to understand relevant concepts and ways of thinking, which can then be incorporated into meaningful behaviours, so including some topics on patient safety in both learning and assessment would seem valuable. A module of learning organized around such topics (see Box 14.1) will ensure that students have a set of working concepts of patient safety, and will raise their awareness of core definitions, the current evidence base for problems and their resolution, and give a theoretical underpinning to their experience of patient safety issues.

Patient safety and assessment

Universities set their own course assessments, while vocational postgraduate programmes may be examined nationally (e.g. Fellowship of the Royal College of Surgeons). Learners tend to prioritize concepts and competencies which are formally assessed in examinations, so this is another argument for making patient safety visible in the learning objectives of the course and its formal assessments. As with other clinical competencies, assessment may be in written format (for knowledge), skills exams (long cases, Objective Structured Clinical Examinations, OSCEs), continuous assessments (clinical placement reports, Record of In-training Assessment, [RITAs]), and formatively through clinical supervision. Bodies such as the accrediting councils are mandated to ensure that assessments (including revalidation) ensure fitness for

---

Box 14.1 A typical undergraduate medical curriculum in patient safety

Key curricular outcome derived from General Medical Council (GMC) guidelines for training doctors[1] – *'Graduates must know about and understand . . . how errors can happen in practice and the principles of managing risk'*

Course covers:

1 Patient scenarios in problem-based learning – prescribing errors, hospital-acquired infection, failure to implement accepted management.
2 Seminar /lectures for theoretical learning:

   (a) Definitions.
   (b) How big is the problem? – epidemiology, the role of reporting systems.
   (c) Analysing the problem – research into patient safety and clinical errors.
   (d) Thinking about error – significant events, root cause analysis, and other ways to learn from errors in clinical settings.
   (e) Tackling the problem – the role of the professional in self-awareness, the team and the environment.
   (f) Systems thinking – ways to prevent and detect risks before they cause harm.

3 Consultation skills practice

   (a) Communication – with colleagues, patients and via information technology.
   (b) Scenarios explaining risks of an operation.
   (c) Scenario with patient's family explaining an error that has occurred.

4 Clinical attachments – reports from tutors regarding safe practice and professional behaviours.

[1] http://www.gmc-uk.org/global_sections/search_frameset.htm

---

purpose, and patient safety is a central policy in this regard, so inclusion of patient safety in assessment would appear to be an important priority. A useful question to focus on is how educators can demonstrate that their learners are coming out as 'safe' practitioners, and where in summative assessments the relevant competencies for safe practice have been assessed.

Linking patient safety to clinical practice

Even when there is a core curriculum of patient safety topics, these will remain a very small component of health professional learners' overall professional development (Howe 2002). It is therefore an educational necessity that clinical placements support the overall curriculum (see Box 14.2). Modern professional training courses in patient safety need to demonstrate a 'safety culture', which is defined by Aron and Headrick (2002) as one which

- acknowledges and learns from error;
- encourages all to improve quality and safety;

Box 14.2 An example of a formal master's module in patient safety[1]

Module outcomes:

- Describe the principles of risk and apply them to health care.
- Critically apply medico-legal principles to their working environment.
- Critically analyse healthcare policy and strategy for managing clinical risk.
- Apply the tools and techniques for identifying, managing and minimizing adverse clinical events.
- Receive, analyse and respond appropriately to complaints about clinical management.
- Communicate information, ideas, problems and solutions relating to clinical risk, to patients and colleagues.

Content:

- Understand adverse incidents, the nature of errors and violations.
- Individual, team and organizational influences on error-producing behaviour.
- Health care as a high-risk enterprise: learning from high reliability organizations.
- Legal principles: law of tort, duty, breach and principles of causation.
- The NHS clinical risk strategy: clinical governance, the role of professional and statutory bodies.
- Assessing, managing and monitoring clinical risk: learning from mistakes, reporting and analysing adverse incidents.
- Managing and learning from complaints.

[1] From MPHe in Population Health Evidence, University of Manchester (http://www.manchester.ac.uk/degreeprogrammes/postgraduate/taught/734.htm).

- is supportive of all personnel to protect patient safety, regardless of rank.

There are some common methods used by clinicians for CPD, which can also be used by learners in clinical placements. These include experiential learning from potential error (Vincent 2003) such as critical event/significant event analysis; methods that develop the learners' skills in systems analysis, such as root cause analysis (see Chapters 8 and 10); and methods that explore clinical reasoning (Dowie and Elstein 1988). Related broader educational approaches into which patient safety can be embedded include consultation and communication skills (Sutcliffe et al. 2004) and problem-based learning.

Sadly, most learners still perceive their peers and seniors to react to potential errors through defensive responses (Aron and Headrick 2002) – the undesirable triad of denial ('it wasn't our fault'), discounting ('it didn't really matter anyway'), and distancing ('what I did wasn't the main cause'). Ideally, those in training will see their clinical teams routinely treat near misses as constructive learning experiences, and will be encouraged by mentors[1] to use these experiences for their own learning. Specialist registrars should receive induction which covers 'Risk Management', both in terms of reporting adverse incidents (reactive) and conducting risk assessments (proactive). More serious adverse incidents gather statements from all relevant staff and are the subject of clinical review, and these may be excellent learning opportunities.[2] Specific learning tools such as portfolios (Mathers et al. 1999) may encourage such reflective practice, and thus enable personal experience to become useful procedural and formal knowledge (Eraut 1994) that can be recurrently of use in practice. Asking learners to debrief significant events in detail will be particularly powerful if combined with formal assessment and personalized feedback to the learners. The use of these approaches in supervisory settings may compensate for any clinical environments which are hostile to such critical enquiry,[3] and the subsequent actions of learners who have become familiar with transparent discussions of adverse events can support policy initiatives that encourage incident reporting and cultural change (NPSA 2003).

Linking patient safety with quality issues

Patient safety is one component of the broader aim of maximizing quality of care, and into this comes learning about clinical governance, evidence-based practice, ethical decision-making, patient-centredness, quality improvement tools including audit (see Chapter 4), and learning about organizations and complex systems. Again, these are likely to be less effective and integrated into practice if they are taught as topics ('did you bother going to that lecture on audit'?) than if they are applied to students' clinical learning and discussed in an interactive setting ('we all had to present our audit projects today and some of the Trust staff came to discuss them'). Quality improvement is an important part of modern practice for all health professionals, and ensuring that placements have learning objectives in these fields will help to 'close the loop' between students perceiving lapses in care and understanding how these can be used to alter care in the future. Ensuring that learners understand the key links between quality, organizational governance, and patient safety is important (see Box 14.2). Effective educational approaches could include 'tracking' an adverse event from their clinical placement through the reporting systems; observing the Patient Advocacy and Liaison staff dealing with patient concerns; or being asked to survey patients for any concerns they may have about their care. Patient voices are often powerful sources of education (Howe and Anderson 2003), so using expert patients as a tutorial resource, or running consultation skills sessions based on scenarios of clinical errors, will focus learners more clearly on the consequences of their actions for patients and their carers.

How have educational approaches been used in patient safety?

Each setting will have considerable variations of opportunity and priority, so the next section is a general outline against which ideas can be checked and options considered. The first consideration is whether there is already a recognizable core curriculum in patient safety, what it includes, and what it omits. Guidance and ideas may be gained from peers elsewhere or from professional bodies such as the Royal Colleges. Nursing and medical peers may know of educational resources or expertise that can assist course and CPD developments, and recent reporting data from Trusts can be useful to highlight contemporary errors affecting patient care.

The second educational approach is supporting learners to debrief clinical experience. Relevant questions include how one ensures this is done rigorously but supportively; looking at the amount of time spent on patient safety issues, including the problems of dealing with poor practice by colleagues: and how clinical mentors deal with these (constructively or defensively? do they ever discuss these things at all?). Useful educational methods include significant event analysis or similar; peer-based learning where students share responsibility for the team's output; patient experiences and concerns; and consultation skills practice with some focus on communicating with colleagues when under pressure, and on explaining errors or adverse events to patients.

A third domain resembles good practice from other industries, and involves the frequent rehearsal of high-risk diagnoses and procedures. Good educational practice requires observation in practice/real life as well as exam conditions, and rigorous assessment of learner competence in these areas.

Finally, there is the need for educational feedback and evaluation. Ex-learners and their employers can be asked for their perceptions of the adequacy of training for patient safety, and ongoing appraisals and CPD opportunities can be used to address patient safety issues (see Box 14.3). Linking personal learning based on significant events with Trust level training and engagement in quality assurance methods makes this 'bite', whereas exercises in ticking boxes and sitting in lecture theatres do not.

Box 14.3 Aspects of CPD approaches to patient safety

- The learner and their professional self-awareness – reflective practice, personal safety netting.
- The learner as a professional practitioner – individual responsibilities.
- The learner and the team – teamwork, mutual awareness, assertiveness.
- The learner and the patient – patient-centred practice, transparency, responsiveness.
- The learner and the educational environment – audit, significant event analysis, error reporting.
- The learner and the organizational culture – risk management, intervening in unsafe practice.

Learner scenarios

The following examples are 'near life' vignettes from people involved with training in patient safety. They are offered as spontaneous quotes to help focus on the realities of clinical learning, and to encourage learner-led developments in patient safety education:

I am on a specialist training scheme in obstetrics and gynaecology. We hold regular perinatal mortality and morbidity meetings where all unexpectedly bad outcomes are reviewed from both the antenatal and neonatal teams in a joint setting. We have guidelines on the management of the common emergencies, and there is a monthly email that highlights any particular problems that may have occurred leading to actual or potentially adverse outcomes. We also have a formal system for reporting adverse events.

There are other more general issues like physical safety – a system of tagging babies and locks on the entrances to labour ward and the ante- and postnatal wards with the use of CCTV. The Trust Induction programme included fire training, particularly with regard to looking after patients during a fire alarm.

I am a consultant paediatrician, and supervise senior house officers and specialist registrars. Their formal induction has a strong clinical governance focus, and includes a session on note keeping using 'mocked up' notes based on real cases. They have to work in groups imagining they are a medico-legal lawyer and go through notes spotting the mistakes. As part of their day release programme, they get teaching on reflective practice, clinical governance and writing up critical incidents. They have to write up at least two critical incidents a year using a specific format, and identify what they have learned from these. Some places have an excellent system of anonymously reviewing all critical incident reports every month which I think should be much more widespread.

In our teaching of allied health professionals, risk assessment is part of induction and the curriculum, and is also considered in placement preparation. This relates to personal risk as a therapist and risk within clinical practice, e.g. patients with challenging behaviours, lone working, equipment and materials. Our teaching on healthcare management addresses clinical governance, fitness for purpose, etc., and always puts patient safety in context of our professional responsibilities and code of conduct.

On practice placements patient safety is a critical component, and forms part of the assessment process. This is related to the specific clinical area – the policies and procedures within each clinical area have to be accessed and understood, and their practice adhered to. Students receive a preparation session which addresses these issues per practice experience, and so develop a clear understanding of their responsibilities.

If students are involved in incidents which compromise patient safety, then we would expect them to follow the procedures of their practice area, but we would follow up any issues of concern reported to tutors with appropriate action. This process is documented as part of our quality assurance mechanism.

In our undergraduate programme, we have to make sure our work on patient safety is replicable over large numbers of students at different sites. We try to incorporate interaction, simulation and reflection, because we think this is a behavioural issue more than just knowing things. We give an overview of examples of major errors, a taxonomy, and look at three types of error – procedures, pre- scribing, and communication. We also look at ethics and team interactions. The big challenge is keeping students alert to this issue in the rest of the course.

I am often struck as a newish student by how difficult it is to know whether someone is doing their job well or not, and then I realize how much patients have to trust us to be doing the right thing. I have seen things that I thought looked dodgy, but then I don't really know whether it matters or not. Once I asked a nurse and she went running off and came back and was cross because everything was OK – that put me off really, I felt stupid, so I probably won't do that again – bother telling someone if I think a bit of equipment isn't working . . . But I like discussing it with tutors because then you can ask questions and make better decisions.

Education – not a 'stand-alone' solution

Organizing effective learning events is a necessary but insufficient means of ensuring that people take on board the tough issues regarding patient safety. Clinical tutors who supervise and mentor health professional learners will know that not all their role models are good, and that the impact of the hidden curriculum – 'those processes, pressures and constraints which fall outside . . . the formal curriculum, and which are often unarticulated or unexplored' (Cribb and Bignold 1999) – can be a much stronger influence in clinical settings than formal teaching. There is a large body of evidence on organizational culture and its influence on behaviour, both for educational and clinical outcomes (Senge 1990). Effective learning needs *both* appropriate curricula *and* a climate whose values and attitudes motivate people to practise safely or otherwise: this involves addressing the general ethos of the clinical environment, which can reinforce or undermine the aims of both formal and experiential learning.

Being motivated to learn requires emotional as well as intellectual engagement, and is significantly influenced by whether learners are operating in a psychologically supportive environment. There are interesting links between psychological defensiveness and poor performance, the conditions for burn-out and the making of inappropriate decisions being closely aligned (Borrell-Carrio and Epstein 2004).

Learners who are not supported to rehearse safe approaches to clinical reasoning and procedural practice may not establish 'hard-wired' cognitive and affective schemata to serve them when under pressure (Nkanginieme 1997), and the ability to challenge self or others requires a degree of self-esteem and/or peer support which must be established in the training environment. This is an explicitly psychological approach, where dealing with uncertainty and concerns is rewarded and encouraged, in order that appropriate responses and values can be internalized and carried into lifelong practice. Contrast this with the shotgun questions and ritual humiliation which are the stuff of some clinical learners' experiences (Lemmp and Seale 2004), and questions arise about whether the necessary conditions exist across clinical settings for students to 'risk' looking at the hard issues regarding patient safety: their own ignorance and uncertainties, challenging seniors, whistle-blowing, and listening to patients (Szauter et al. 2003). If this is not consistently part of their learning as students, it is unlikely that they will establish habits of transparency and constructive criticism in post-training settings.

Another part of the learning environment is learning teamwork. This will be dealt with in more detail in Chapter 16 by Pearce et al., but is mentioned here because peers are a very strong influence in vocational courses, especially in postgraduate practice where staff still in training may supervise other learners, and in courses using problem-based learning where the peer group is a major educational resource. Again, education for patient safety needs both to be visible and valued in the peer setting, and those in more senior positions need to understand how influential they are on junior staff, and to be motivated to explore these issues and model appropriate responses wherever possible.

Cultural change and educational reform

Many involved in education are clearer about what they would want to do than how to get there, and the parallels between factors producing change in education or clinical practice are considerable. Cultural change can be produced by shifting the balance of power from staff to patients (Davies et al. 2000), which is part of the rationale for early and repeated patient contact during training; and encouraging collaboration rather than competition among peers, for example, through shared learning. Cultural transformation can also be supported by outside influences (such as the requirements of accrediting bodies and key national agencies), policy imperatives, and keen opinion leaders who champion the educational themes concerned. Clinical staff who care passionately about patient safety and who are inspiring teachers and local opinion leaders can be crucial in this regard. Staff development through a core of committed tutors will ensure that the preferred learning culture of a course has been portrayed to the clinical mentors, and this can support patient safety learning from practice.

Learning with others is another strong source of influence on learner awareness of patient safety issues. Different disciplines have very different priorities in this regard, with surgical teams and theatre-based staff being very aware of technical aspects, pharmacy leading on issues around medicines safety, nursing being relatively procedurally oriented and using team support effectively for safety netting, while doctors are more autonomous and have the whole scope of patient care under their remit. Issues of inter-professional communication, barriers to effective co-operation, and best use of shared records are just a few examples of issues which cannot be fully addressed in a uni-disciplinary learning environment. Again, the clinical setting provides many opportunities for shared learning, but these can only be effective if the team takes time to explore them as a multidisciplinary group – an approach which is explored more fully in Chapter 16.

Future challenges

This brief summary is designed to stimulate thought and ideas on improving education for health professionals. It shows that involvement in clinical learning and day-to-day critical enquiry in practice is seen as a key learning method by both students and tutors, and having an environment of open discussion and reporting is vital. Even if this is not consistently provided across all learning settings, it seems that each training scheme should provide something where patient safety can be safely and fully debriefed, and a formal curriculum can complement this by giving conceptual frameworks and putting the issues 'on the agenda'. There is a reasonable consensus as to areas to be covered, but a defensive organizational culture will make this kind of learning more difficult, as will didactic methods and lack of detailed clinical supervision. The links with communication, quality and teamwork must be made explicit, and the conditions under which good practice begins to break down needs to be very familiar to our learners, so that their conscious warning bells are set off before errors occur. To help our learners learn from mistakes, tutors must be prepared to make their own experiences of risk a subject of legitimate enquiry. Patient safety is a topic for a new kind of learning – one that puts the patient first, the learner second, our failures in the open, and our humility to the test. This is what we can really call a learning culture.

Notes

1   The mentoring role may be various titled supervisor, personal tutor or adviser, mentor, trainer – its meaning in this chapter is the person whose main role is to assist professional development by helping the student to learn from clinical experiences.
2   M. Davies, personal communication.
3   D. Bowman, personal communication.

Box 14.4 Key points

• Patient safety should be taught as part of the formal curriculum for the training of health professionals.
• Patient safety should also form part of formal assessment for health professionals.
• Patient safety needs to be part of the training culture as well as the formal process if the training is to achieve its aims.
• Culture change can be achieved by shifting the balance of power to patients, outside influences, policy imperatives and opinion leaders, as well as learning with and from others.
• Relevant educational methods including learning from experience of adverse events and training in quality improvement, using innovative methods such as patient tracking and listening to the voice of the patient.
• Learning is affected by emotional engagement, and psychological issues are important here, as is learning how to work effectively in teams.
• Each training programme should encourage an understanding of patient safety, within a supportive culture, and links to other aspects of learning must be acknowledged.
• Patient safety is a topic for a new kind of learning – one that puts the patient first, the learner second, our failures in the open, and our humility to the test – a true 'learning culture'.

References

Aron, D.C. and Headrick, L.A. (2002) Educating physicians to improve care and safety is no accident: it requires a systematic approach. *Quality and Safety in Health Care*, 11: 168–73.

Borrell-Carrio, F. and Epstein, R. (2004) Preventing errors in clinical practice: a call for self awareness. *Annals of Family Medicine*, 2: 310–16.

Brennan, T.A. (2002) Physicians' professional responsibility to improve the quality of care, *Academic Medicine*, 77(10): 973–80.

Cribb, A. and Bignold, S. (1999) Towards the reflexive medical school: the hidden curriculum and medical education research, *Studies in Higher Education*, 24(2): 195–209.

Davies, H.T.O., Nutley, S. and Mannion, R. (2000) Organizational culture and quality of health care, *Quality and Safety in Health Care*, 9: 111–19.

Dowie, J. and Elstein, A. (eds) (1988) *Professional Judgement: A Reader in Clinical Decision-Making*. Cambridge: Cambridge University Press.

Eraut, M. (1994) *Developing Professional Knowledge and Competence*. London: Falmer Press.

Howe, A. (2002) Professional development in undergraduate medical curricula: the key to the door of a new culture? *Medical Education*, 36(4): 353–9.

Howe, A. and Anderson, J. (2003) Learning in practice: involving patients in medical education, *British Medical Journal*, 327: 326–8.

Lempp, H. and Seale, C. (2004) The hidden curriculum in undergraduate medical education: qualitative study of medical students' perceptions of teaching. *British Medical Journal*, 329: 770–3.

Mathers, N.J., Challis, M., Howe, A. and Field, N.J. (1999) Portfolios in continuing medical education: effective and efficient? *Medical Education*, 33(7): 521–53.

National Patient Safety Agency (2003) *Seven Steps to Patient Safety: A Guide for NHS Staff*. London: NPSA.

Nkanginieme, K. (1997) Clinical diagnosis as a dynamic cognitive process: application of Bloom's taxonomy for educational objectives in the cognitive domain. *Med Educ Online* 2:1. Available from: http://www.Med-Ed-Online

Senge, P.M. (1990) *The Fifth Discipline: The Art and Practice of the Learning Organization*. New York: Doubleday.

Sutcliffe, K.M., Lewton, E. and Rosenthal, M.M. (2004) Communication failures: an insidious contribution to medical mishaps, *Academic Medicine*, 79(2): 189–94.

Szauter, K., Williams, B., Ainsworth, M.A., Callaway, M., Bulik, R. and Camp, M.G. (2003) Student perceptions of professional behaviour of faculty physicians. *Med Educ Online* 8:17. Available from http://www.Med-Ed-Online

Vincent, C. (2003) Patient safety: understanding and responding to adverse events, *New England Journal of Medicine*, 348: 1051–6.

15

Pathways to patient safety
The use of rules and guidelines in health care
Tanya Claridge, Dianne Parker and Gary Cook

Using rules to manage quality and safety

One of the key features of organized society is the development of a system of social rules and behavioural norms. The principal functions of such systems are to reflect societal and cultural values, and to safeguard things of value. Rules come in many different forms, including conventions, laws and social norms. Fukuyama (2000) has suggested that rules may be formal or informal, and permissive or restrictive. In addition, there are regulative rules, which regulate naturally occurring behaviour and constitutive rules, which relate to the structure of a system and the exercise of power and influence within that system. Thus, rules of etiquette are regulative because they seek to regulate social interactions, whereas laws are constitutive as they enforce rules designed to maintain the social order. Some rules are based on fundamental moral principles (it is wrong to commit murder), while others serve as a form of social control, prescribing anti-social behaviour (it is wrong to drop litter). Many rules exist purely in order to ensure that social affairs run smoothly. For example, driving on the right-hand side of the road is not intrinsically safer than driving on the left, but in many countries there is a rule (in this case, with the force of law) that all drivers will keep to the right. This rule has been imposed as a way of introducing standardization and increasing predictability in a complex system.

In the social psychological literature, three motives for obeying rules have been distinguished (Tyler 1990). People may obey a rule because they believe that the rule-maker has legitimate authority in the area, because they feel that breaking the rule would lead to negative consequences for them, or because they see that the rule is fair and is applied in a fair and equitable manner. This last motive is often under-estimated by rule-makers, who assume that the imposition of ever-harsher punishments for transgressions is the best way to increase rule compliance. In fact, the likelihood that a rule will be obeyed is more strongly linked to the perception that it is a fair rule (Tyler 1990).

The development and implementation of rules are one of the most common ways to manage behaviour in complex organizations (Hopwood 1974). The promotion of safety is one area of organizational behaviour in which rules feature heavily. Reason's

(1995) model of organizational safety indicates that rules, in the form of procedures, protocols and guidelines are one of the principal defences necessary to ensure a safe organization. However, rules cannot work as a means of ensuring safety unless they are known, understood and complied with by all those expected to work to them.

In developing and implementing safety rules, organizations tend to make the assumption that the rules are good ones and that they will be followed. For example, there are many rules governing the use of personal protective equipment (PPE) in hazardous industrial contexts, in order to protect workers' heads, eyes, hands and feet. Typically, managers provide this equipment, explain its purpose, and confidently expect employees to use it at all times. In fact, accident analysis has shown that rule-breaking behaviour is a common problem in the context of organizational safety (McDonald et al. 2000). Subsequently, researchers have investigated the reasons for non-compliance with safety rules (Reason et al. 1994; Hudson et al. 1998; Dimmer 2001). Many organizational factors have been identified as potential explanations of non-compliance with rules. These include the imposition of a higher priority on production and less on security (Reason 1997); problems with rules and feedback affecting perceptions of personal gains and losses (Battmann and Klumb 1993), conflicts between personal and organizational goals (Reason et al. 1998) and a perceived lack of risk in failing to comply with the rule (Zeitlin 1994; Gonzalea and Sawicka 2002). In the context of the UK National Health Service, the current emphasis on standards and targets (especially targets related to process, for instance, waiting times) may result in a distortion of clinical priorities. This could result in the care provided being driven according to political targets, not evidence-based practice, thus undermining the safety of patients, a view echoed by politicians, clinicians and academics (Miller 2003; Yeo 2004; Mannion et al. 2005).

The distinction between error and violation is important in this context (see Chapter 3) because these different types of rule-breaking demand different remedies. Errors occur when the safety rule is not known or is forgotten. For example, an operator may fail to appreciate the need to wear a hard hat on site at all times. Errors can best be reduced by interventions designed to optimize the deployment of attentional resources, for example, training or the use of reminders. Violations, on the other hand, are intentional and, in terms of safety, reflect risk-taking behaviour. In this case, the failure to put on a hard hat would be a conscious decision to break a known safety rule. Neither training nor the provision of reminders would be likely to have an effect in that situation. The key to reducing the violation of safety rules is to persuade perpetrators not to commit them (Parker et al. 1995, 1996).

In the context of reducing the violation of safety procedures in the oil and gas industry Hudson et al. (1998) produced a list of steps that must be taken in order to maximize compliance. First, the organization should review all existing rules and ensure that they are correct, comprehensible and available to employees and understood by them. Second, any unnecessary, out-of-date or unworkable procedures should be revised or abandoned. Third, the organization should ensure that compliance with the remaining procedures is actually possible. This means providing the training, equipment and time necessary for full compliance. Fourth, any factors that encourage the violation of rules must be eliminated. For example, it must be ensured that the time saved by failing to follow a safety procedure does not 'earn' employees any benefit, for example, an extra coffee break. At the same time, organizations must acknowledge that it is not possible to develop a rule to cover every possible situation. Attempting to do so will almost certainly lead to the stifling of initiative, and produce employees who do not know how to react when a novel situation arises (Hale 1990).

Using rules to improve patient safety in health care

The use of rules or protocols in health care is not a new phenomenon. Semi-formal and formal rules in various guises have been used for a number of years in all sectors of health care to regulate safety-critical ancillary activities, for instance, storage of controlled and prescription drugs (Yee 1998) and hand washing (McCarthy et al. 1993). They have also been used with reference to the actual delivery of clinical care, for instance, guidelines on clinical technique and history taking are often presented in handbooks on clerking patients in (Swash and Hutchinson 2001), and within the nursing process (Roper et al. 1983). However, in recent years national healthcare policy has begun to focus on the use of rules specifically as a way of managing quality and safety.

The implementation of EBP (Evidence Based Practice) is one area in which rules have been used as the vehicle for improving quality. Previously, even when clinical effectiveness was supported by apparently rigorous evidence, this proved insufficient to produce related changes in practice. For example, Schuster et al. (1998) postulated that 30–40 per cent patients do not get treatment of proven effectiveness and 20–25 per cent patients get care that is not needed or is potentially harmful (Schuster et al. 1998). In response to the slow pace of progress towards EBP, policy interest increased in the use of rules to promote the use of evidence-based practice (Grol 1991). For instance, the UK NHS Plan (Department of Health 2000b) specified that 'by 2004 the majority of NHS staff will be working under agreed protocols' and that there will be 'a major drive to ensure that protocol based care takes hold throughout the NHS'.

In terms of patient safety, there is also a move internationally towards the use of rules to regulate the behaviour of healthcare professionals (Kohn et al. 2000). In 2002, a World Alliance for Patient Safety was formed, and has passed a resolution urging the World Health Organization to take the lead in developing global norms and standards. The assumption is that, as in other high-risk industries, patient safety can be improved by increasing standardization and predictability in the system. In the UK, one of the recommendations of the Department of Health report, *Organization with a Memory*, was that 'consideration should be given to the production and piloting of standardised procedural manuals and safety bulletins which it is obligatory to use when embarking on specific high risk procedures' (2000a: 86).

The drive for the implementation of EBP, coupled with increased awareness of patient safety issues in recent years, has seen a proliferation of formal (active) or semi-formal (passive) rules, developed in order to standardize and manage the behaviour of healthcare professionals. The most common type of rule in health care is a protocol, which is essentially a set of instructions that can be formatted in a variety of different ways and used in many different clinical contexts. Passive protocols (Coiera 2003), for instance, guidelines, are semi-formal. They do not direct patient management, but provide guidance and add to the information resources available. Passive protocols are accessed or used at the discretion of the healthcare professional. In contrast, active or formal protocols (for instance, Integrated Care Pathways, known as ICPs) are prescriptive, actively managing patient care in some way. Active protocols are fundamentally different to passive protocols, in that they are central to the way the patient is managed, rather than an optional accessory. The way protocols are formatted also varies. Active protocols can be computer-based and include alerts when there is deviation from the protocol (e.g. GP prescribing software). However, the majority of active protocols are paper-based, allowing their effect on actual practice to be evaluated through audit.

Protocols, in any format, are seen by their exponents as 'tools that ensure service development is driven by evidence of clinical or cost effectiveness, for improving the safety of and consistency of care, and for co-ordinating health services' (Dillon and Hargadon 2003). In other words, protocols are educational tools that lead to improvements in the quality of care and in patient safety. Unfortunately, there is some evidence that the proliferation of rules of different types has led to confusion among healthcare professionals about the differential status and functions of rules, procedures, guidelines and protocols in health care. Claridge, Parker and Cook's study (2001, 2005) showed that the difference between an active (formal) protocol and a passive (informal) protocol was not clearly understood, and that the confusion was compounded when both were contained within a single Integrated Care Pathway.

It is clear that in health care, as in other organizational settings, merely having guidelines and protocols in place is not sufficient to improve safety (Reason 1997; Goldberg et al. 1998; Lawton and Parker 1998; Shaneyfelt et al. 1999). Even when protocols are readily available, healthcare professionals have been shown to forget to follow them or deviate from them without a clear reason (Claridge et al. 2001). To have an effect, rules have to be followed. Research from all sectors of health care in the UK and world-wide suggests that this is not often the case (European Secondary Prevention Study Group 1996; Halm et al. 2000; van Wijk et al. 2001).

While this research demonstrates that guidelines are not always adhered to, it does not necessarily indicate why. Much of the research considering the behaviour of healthcare professionals in relation to the implementation of ICPs, guidelines or other forms of rules in health care has focussed on the attributes of the guidelines themselves. For instance, a study by Durieux et al. (2000) showed a change in doctor behaviour and improved compliance with guidelines following the introduction of a Clinical Decision Support System for the prevention of venous thrombo-embolism.

A less conventional, but maybe more useful, approach is one that considers what it is about rules that healthcare professionals don't seem to like. Lawton and Parker (1998) used focus groups to investigate the attitudes of doctors to protocols and found that they felt that the complex and unpredictable nature of their work does not lend itself to the 'straitjacket' effect of them on clinical practice.

It is crucial that rules in health care such as ICPs, designed to influence and control behaviour, are both understood and accepted by those expected to use them. We have undertaken a programme of research that investigated the attitudes of healthcare professionals towards Integrated Care Pathways specifically, using interviews, focus group discussions and surveys (Claridge et al. 2001, 2005). One of the aims was to ascertain what healthcare professionals see as the main problem with ICPs. A questionnaire survey of 246 healthcare professionals was used to ascertain views about the prescription of clinical practice, the evidence base contained in ICPs, and the format of the documentation. We wanted to find out whether the real problem, from the perspective of those expected to use them, is the idea, the content or the form of ICPs.

In one study the aspect that attracted the most negative ratings reflected the function of ICPs in structuring healthcare professionals' practice. The survey covered doctors, nurses and PAMs. All three groups felt that ICPs were designed to control their practice, taking away their ability to use their professional autonomy when dealing with patients and leading to a lack of individualized patient care. This finding was confirmed in a subsequent multi-site survey of the attitudes of healthcare professionals (n = 375) towards ICPs, (Claridge 2005) and is supported by the findings of other research and reviews (Dowsell et al. 2001; Timmermans and Mauck 2005). Again, when respondents were asked to rate different sources of dissatisfaction with the implementation and use of ICPs, the structuring of health care in general was the most important one. Figure 15.1 depicts the findings.

Strengths and weaknesses of using rules to improve patient safety

The findings of this study have important implications for those charged with the development and implementation of ICPs or with structuring the delivery of health care in general using protocol-based care. In spite of the fact that, anecdotally, many people grumbled about the format of the documents themselves, our analyses suggested that staff actually had more problems with the whole concept of ICPs than with either their format or their content. This suggests that investing time and effort in changing the presentation of ICPs will not meet with success until more fundamental aspects of staff unease have been addressed. The healthcare professionals involved in

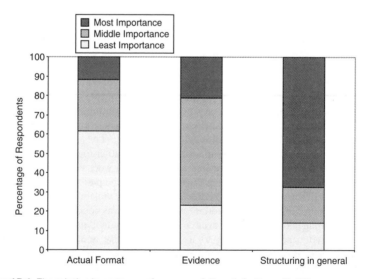

Figure 15.1 The relative importance of sources of dissatisfaction with ICPs

these studies were negative about ICP use because they did not like the idea of being told what to do. While the general approach of using rules to standardize and regulate behaviour can be successful, these findings indicate that the ICP development programme will fail unless the hearts and minds of those expected to use ICPs have been won over. The implementation process, as it stands, appears not to consider this issue, with the result that chances of success in improving patient safety are compromised.

Further analysis of the data revealed that junior healthcare professionals, whether they were doctors, nurses or PAMs, tended to have a significantly less positive attitude towards ICPs than their more senior counterparts. This seemingly counter-intuitive finding may reflect the fact that senior staff do not feel that ICPs actually apply to them, and so do not feel threatened in the same way. They see ICPs as a way of regulating the behaviour of juniors, but not their own. Alternatively, it may be that junior staff dislike ICPs more than senior staff do because they are at a stage in their career when they are most keen to exercise professional judgement and to put into practice all they have learned relatively recently. This group may feel that they are now fully qualified professionals and have left behind training, so may be somewhat dismayed to find that they are expected to complete 'tick box exercises' and to justify their practice on a daily basis.

Again, if either of these two speculative explanations are correct, then more education and explanation of the rationale behind the introduction of ICPs and protocol-based care is necessary, in order to win the approval of junior clinicians. They must be informed about why ICPs are felt to be necessary, and the importance of complying with them, both in terms of completing the documentation and in terms of using them to guide practice. Currently, this represents a further area of weakness in the general approach.

It is also important to know whether the widespread non-compliance with guidelines that has been noted (Grol et al. 1998), is the result of genuine error or of deliberate decisions on the part of the individual. To date, the distinction between error and violation has been generally neglected in terms of medical error (Dovey et al. 2002). We investigated this issue by asking 246 healthcare professionals to judge the behaviour of a colleague as described in hypothetical scenarios (Parker et al. 2005). The content of the scenarios was experimentally manipulated so that the same rule-breaking behaviour was presented as either an error or a violation.

The results of this survey indicated widespread resentment of the use of ICPs as a form of administrative control, especially among doctors, who saw them as a challenge to the self-regulation traditional in medicine. The judgement of doctors appeared to be driven by the outcome for the patient rather than the characteristics of the behaviour of the healthcare professional. Doctors were not likely to disapprove of the violation of an ICP providing the outcome for the patient was a good one. On the other hand, nurses were less comfortable with rule violations and disapproved of non-compliance whether the outcome for the patient was good, poor or bad.

In summary, the impetus towards the development and implementation of protocol-based care as a means to improving quality and safety appears to be gathering pace. Both nationally and internationally, a great deal of importance in health care is being attached to the development and implementation of rules, often in the form of protocols, case management tools or ICPs.

Future challenges

Explanatory frameworks and/or models from social science and high-risk industry are potentially useful in considering, understanding and explaining rule-related behaviour of healthcare professionals. In order to ensure the success of protocol-based care as a way of managing safety, it is imperative that the lessons learned from experience in other high-risk industries are taken into account.

For rules to be followed they must be appropriate, and as simple and easy to apply as possible. Given the complexities of modern health care, it must be accepted that it will not always be feasible to develop a protocol prescribing the correct course of action ahead of time. It is also important to acknowledge that conditions at the patient interface may make it difficult or impossible to access and apply the relevant protocol appropriately.

The implementation of protocol-based care requires careful management if compliance levels are to be improved. At the moment, they are often seen as a back-covering exercise, and/or an unnecessary administrative burden. The implementation of protocol-based care without educating and resourcing the healthcare professionals expected to follow the protocols is unlikely to lead to success.

There is also a need for healthcare professionals to be clear about the status and function of protocol-based care. In order to address this issue, the use of protocols to manage patient care needs to be situated clearly as a high priority within the organization, perhaps by giving a high-level management group overall responsibility for the development and implementation processes. This level of formal management commitment may be necessary to drive a protocol-based care programme if it is to be accepted and successful among staff at all levels. It is essential that protocol-based care is not perceived as yet another initiative dreamed up centrally and imposed on an already overstretched workforce with insufficient consultation.

Box 15.1 Key points

- There is an international move towards the use of rules in health care to manage patient safety.
- Protocol-based care embodies the use of guidelines, protocols, care plans and Integrated Care Pathways, these are all types of rule.
- Such rules may cover the delivery of care directly, the ancillary processes that surround care delivery, or both.
- Many lessons can be learned from other high-risk industries on how to develop and implement rules in order to maximize compliance.
- There is evidence that healthcare professionals are uncertain of the status and function of the rules that they are expected to follow.
- There is also evidence that healthcare professionals are not comfortable with the care that they deliver being structured by rules.
- The development and implementation of protocol-based care in health care require very careful management if they are to be successful and contribute to the safety of patients.

References

Battmann, W. and Klumb, P. (1993) Behavioural economics and compliance with safety regulations, *Safety Science*, 16(1): 35–46.

Campbell, H., Hotchkiss, R., Bradshaw, N. and Porteous, M. (1998) Integrated care pathways, *British Medical Journal*, 316(7125): 133–7.

Claridge, T. (2005) Human Facts, Human Error and Health Care Professionals (unpublished doctors thesis).

Claridge, T., Parker, D. and Cook, G. (2001) The attitudes of health care professionals towards Integrated Care Pathways. In Stockport NHS Trust, *An Investigation: Report to Stockport NHS Trust*. Stockport: Stockport NHS Trust.

Claridge, T., Parker, D. and Cook, G. (2005) Investigating the attitudes of health care professionals towards SCPs, a discussion study, *Journal of Integrated Care Pathways*, 9: 1–10 (in press).

Coiera, E. (2003) *Guide to Health Informatics*. London: Hodder Arnold.

Department of Health (2000a) *Organization with a Memory*. London: The Stationery Office.

Department of Health (2000b) *The NHS Plan*. London: The Stationery Office.

Department of Health (2001) *Protocol Based Care*. London: The Stationery Office.

Dillon, A. and Hargadon, J. (2003) In Modernisation Agency and NICE, Protocol Based Care. Available at http://www.modern.nhs.uk/protocolbasedcare/ (accessed 3 January 2005).

Dimmer, A. (2001) An investigation into the attitudes, driving violations and road accidents of company car drivers, unpublished PhD thesis, University of Manchester.

Dovey, S.M., Meyers, D.S., Phillips, R.L., Green, L.A., Fryer, G.E., Galliher, J.M., Kappus, J. and Grob, P. (2002) A preliminary taxonomy of medical errors in family practice, *Quality and Safety in Health Care*, 11: 23–8.

Dowsell, G., Harrison, S. and Wright, J. (2001) Clinical guidelines: attitudes, information processes and culture in English primary care, *The International Journal of Health Planning and Management*, 16(2): 107–34.

Durieux, P., Nizard, R., Ravaud, P., Mounier, N. and Lepage, E. (2000) A clinical decision support system for prevention of venous thromboembolism effect on physician behavior, *Journal of the American Medical Association*, 283: 2816–21.

European Secondary Prevention Group (1996) Translation of clinical trials into practice: a European population-based study of the use of thrombolysis for acute myocardial infarction, *Lancet*, 347: 1203–7.

Fukuyama, F. (2000) *The Great Disruption: Human Nature and the Deconstitution of Social Order*. London: Profile Books.

Goldberg, H.I., Wagner, E.H., Fihn, S.D., Martin, D.P., Horowitz, C.R., Christensen, D.B., Cheadle, A.D., Diehr, P. and Simon, G. (1998) A randomized control trial of CQI teams and academic detailing: can they alter compliance with guidelines? *Joint Commission Journal on Quality Improvement*, 24: 130–42.

Gonzalez, J.J. and Sawicka, A. (2002) A framework for human factors in information security, in *Proceedings of the 2002 WSEAS International Conference on Information Security (ICIS'02)*. WSEAS.

Grol, R. (2001) Successes and failures in the implementation of evidence-based guidelines for clinical practice, *Medical Care*, 39(8): 46–54.

Grol, R., Dalhuijsen, J., Thomas, S., in 't Veld, C., Rutten, H. and Mokkink, H. (1998) Attributes of clinical guidelines that influence use of guidelines in general practice: observational study, *British Medical Journal*, 317: 858–61.

Hale, A. (1990) Safety rules OK? Possibilities and limitations in behavioural safety strategies, *Journal of Occupational Accidents*, 12: 3–20.

Halm, E., Atlas, S., Borowsky, L., Benzer, T., Metlay, J., Chang, Y. and Singer, D. (2000) Understanding physician behaviour with a pneumonia practice guideline, *Archives of Internal Medicine*, 160: 98–104.

Hopwood, A.G. (1974) *Accounting Systems and Management Behaviour.* Farnborough: Saxon House.

Hudson, P.T.W., Verschuur, W.L.G., Lawton, R.L., Parker, D. and Reason, J.T. (1998) *Bending the Rules II: Why Do People Break Rules or Fail to Follow Procedures, and What Can You Do About It?* the Hague: Shell SIEP.

Kohn, L., Corrigan, J. and Donaldson, M. (eds) (2000) *To Err Is Human: Building a Safer Health System.* Washington, DC: National Academy Press.

Lawton, R.L. and Parker, D. (1998) Procedures and the professional: the case of the British NHS, *Risk Decision and Policy*, 3: 199–211.

Lawton, R.L. and Parker, D. (2002) Judgements of rule-related behaviour in health care professionals: an experimental study, *British Journal of Health Psychology*, 7: 253–65.

Mannion, R., Davies, H. and Marshall, M. (2005) Impact of star performance ratings in English acute hospital trusts, *Journal of Health Service Research and Policy*, 10(1): 18–24.

McCarthy, G.M., Koval, J.J. and MacDonald, J.K. (1999) Compliance with recommended infection control procedures among Canadian dentists: results of a national survey, *American Journal of Infection Control*, 5: 377–84.

McDonald, N., Corrigan, S., Daly, C. and Cromie, S. (2000) Safety management systems and safety culture in aircraft maintenance, *Safety Science*, 34: 151–76.

Miller, P. (2003) Speech to the consultant's conference. Available at http://www.bma.org.uk/ap.nsf/Content/CCSCconf03sp (accessed 3 January 2005).

Modernisation Agency and NICE (2003) *Protocol Based Care.* London: The Stationery Office. Available at http://www.modern.nhs.uk/protocolbasedcare/ (accessed 3 January 2005).

Parker, D., Claridge. T. and Cook, G. (2005) Attitudes towards integrated care pathways in the UK NHS. *Journal of Integrated Care Pathways*, 9: 13–20.

Parker, D. and Lawton, R.L. (2000) Judging the use of clinical protocols by fellow professionals, *Social Science and Medicine*, 51: 669–77.

Parker, D., Manstead, A.S.R. and Stradling, S.G. (1996) Modifying beliefs and attitudes to exceeding the speed limit: an intervention study based on the theory of planned behaviour, *Journal of Applied Social Psychology*, 26: 1–19.

Parker, D., West, R.W., Stradling, S.G. and Manstead, A.S.R. (1995) Behavioural characteristics and involvement in different types of road traffic accident, *Accident Analysis and Prevention*, 27: 571–81.

Reason, J. (1995) A systems approach to organizational error, *Ergonomics*, 38: 1708–21.

Reason, J. (1997) *Managing the Risks of Organizational Accidents.* Brookfield, VE: Ashgate.

Reason, J., Manstead, A., Stradling, S., Baxter, J. and Campbell, K. (1990) Errors and violations: a real distinction? *Ergonomics*, 33: 1315–32.

Reason, J., Parker, D. and Free, R.J. (1994) *Bending the Rules: The Varieties, Origins and Management of Safety Violations.* Report to Shell SIEP, the Hague, September 1994.

Reason, J., Parker, D. and Lawton, R. (1998) Organizational controls and safety: the varieties of rule related behaviour, *Journal of Occupational and Organizational Psychology*, 71: 289–304.

Roper, N., Logan, W. and Tierney, A. (eds) (1983) *Using a Model for Nursing.* Edinburgh: Churchill Livingstone.

Schuster, M.A., McGlynn, E.A. and Brook, R.H. (1998) How good is health care in the United States? *Milbank Quarterly*, 76: 517–63.

Shaneyfelt, T.M., Mayo-Smith, M.F. and Rothwangl, J. (1999) Are guidelines following guidelines? The methodological quality of clinical practice guidelines in the peer-reviewed medical literature, *Journal of the American Medical Association*, 281: 1900–5.

Swash, M. (ed.) (2001) *Hutchinson's Clinical Methods*. 21st edn. London: WB Saunders.

Timmermans, S. and Mauck, A. (2005) The promises and pitfalls of evidence-based medicine, *Health Affairs*, 24(1): 18–28.

Tyler, T. (1990) *Why People Obey the Law*. New Haven, CT: Yale University Press.

Van Wijk, M., van der Lei, J., Mosseveld, M., Bohnen, A. and van Bemmel, J. (2001) Assessment of decision support for blood test ordering in primary care, *Annals of Internal Medicine*, 134(4): 274–81.

Wallace, L.M., Freeman, T., Latham, L., Walshe, K. and Spurgeon, P. (2001) Organizational strategies for changing clinical practice: how trusts are meeting the challenges of clinical governance, *Quality in Health Care*, 10: 76–82.

Yee, S.K. (1998) What you need to know: guidelines to medical practitioners for proper maintenance of drugs and dispensing records (including controlled drugs), *Singapore Medical Journal*, 39(11): 520–2.

Yeo, T. (2004) The health of the NHS: targets distort clinical priorities. Available at www.politics.co.uk (accessed 22 February 2005).

Zeitlin, L.R. (1994) Failure to follow safety instructions: faulty communication or risky decisions? *Human Factors*, 36: 172–81.

16

Team performance, communication and patient safety

Shirley Pearce, Fiona Watts and Alison Watkin

The report *An Organization with a Memory* (Department of Health 2000a) from the Chief Medical Officer arose from the growing recognition that the NHS could no longer continue to ignore the fact that staff involved in patient care may make errors which puts the safety of patients at risk. Much of the focus of the early considerations of clinical errors and mistakes has been directed at the medical profession and the errors and risks associated with surgery and medication.

Clearly, surgeons and physicians, through their actions, can perform direct life-saving or life-threatening tasks and we need to know the influences on their performance that can lead to an intervention or clinical decision being 'faulty' or risk-enhancing as opposed to risk-reducing for the patient receiving that intervention.

But clinical care is not delivered by doctors alone. Health care is delivered by groups of people drawn from a range of professions in combination with a range of different support staff. An adverse outcome for the patient can potentially be 'caused' by errors by any members of this group, not just the medical staff, even though they often take overall legal responsibility for the patient's outcome.

Understanding the influences on medical errors as a way of improving patient safety is clearly important but in view of the complexity of healthcare delivery, it is likely to be only one part of the jigsaw in terms of what needs to be done to maximize patient safety.

This chapter turns the attention to team functioning as one of the factors that influences patient safety and patient outcomes. Whoever is legally responsible for the patient's overall safety, from the patient's perspective, care is delivered by a large number of people who operate together. This group may include the receptionist/ward clerk who greets them and gives them information, the anaesthetist who puts them to sleep, the surgeon who operates, the nurse who supervises their recovery, the physiotherapist who helps in the rehabilitation to the occupational therapist who helps the patient adjust to daily living. The patient perceives their treatment as delivered by this, more or less, coherent and integrated group of staff. And these are just the staff that the patient sees. Behind the scenes are large numbers of technicians and support staff who contribute to the patient's safety by, for example, ordering the right supplies, maintaining equipment safely, or preparing and sorting drugs efficiently. All of these people can make performance errors that can affect patient safety. It also follows that inadequate communication between members of these groups can lead to an adverse outcome, even if each individual's performance as judged on its own may not constitute an 'error'. It is this recognition of the importance of team functioning in healthcare delivery that has led to an interest in how healthcare teams work and what can be done to improve their performance.

The NHS Plan (Department of Health 2000b) was explicit in identifying teamworking as something that should be improved and respected. In addition, it acknowledged 'old-fashioned demarcations' between the health professions and identified these as a significant constraint on improvement and efficiency in the modern NHS. This focus on improving teamworking and communication in the delivery of care has had a significant impact on the education of healthcare professionals. As a consequence, most UK higher education institutions now include some specific educational experiences that improve students' understanding of other professionals and the factors that influence effective teamworking, as part of their pre-registration training programmes.

The speed with which educational establishments are responding to the call to teach teamworking skills and offer interprofessional learning in pre-registration training is, however, somewhat at odds with the relative lack of progress at improving teamworking within the NHS among already qualified staff. This is perhaps not surprising given the largely uni-professional basis for continuing professional development (CPD) in the health professions and the real constraints to achieving change in working practices.

In this chapter we shall first of all review the evidence that team functioning is related to the quality of patient outcomes and hence patient safety. We will then consider ways in which team functioning in the clinical environment might be improved and consider some of the constraints on its efficacy. Finally, we will suggest that team functioning might be considered as a legitimate part of the performance management process of an organization so as to ensure that improvement in team functioning following any particular intervention is maintained and consolidated as part of normal, routine practice.

What is a team?

There are a number of different definitions of the term team. A typical example is that of Baguley (2002) who states that a team is a 'group of people who work together towards a shared and meaningful outcome in ways that combine their individual skills and abilities and for which they are all responsible'. West and Slater (1996) suggest that teams have the following characteristics:

- a collective responsibility for achieving shared aims and objectives;
- an interactive approach among members in order to achieve these objectives;
- more or less defined roles for each individual member, at least some of which are differentiated from each other;
- a team identity.

Implicit in these definitions is the fact that different team members bring different skills/knowledge to the management of a shared problem. Hence, for teams to work at their best, all members must understand what the skills and potential contributions of each of their colleagues are. They must also embrace the importance of effective communication in order to bring all these different attributes to bear in the solution/ management of the shared task.

Clinical case management is an excellent example of teamworking where a range of different sets of skills are required to provide all-round care for the patient. It seems obvious that the patient will receive the best care when all team members are best supported to deliver their particular expertise in a fully co-ordinated way with each other. However, anecdotal evidence suggests this is not always the case and care is often not well co-ordinated, with professionals failing to understand the full benefits of each other's skills.

Even in clinical settings where teamworking is at its most explicit, for example, in operating theatres where surgeons, nurses, anaesthetists and others are working in the same location and in contact with the patient at the same time, the quality of teamworking has been questioned. Silén-Lipponen et al. (2005) describe a qualitative analysis of nurses' views of the sources of error in an operating theatre environment. They conclude that poor teamworking skills are a major source of error and identify four contributing factors to poor teamworking. These are: (1) fear of errors (and humiliation); (2) turnover in teams (and associated lack of knowledge of each team members' skills); (3) overtime pressures (led by some professionals); and (4) emotional distress (hostile behaviour, lack of respect). They argue that improvements to the quality of teamwork would lead to improvements in patient safety.

A further complication is that there are many different kinds of teams in healthcare settings – in GP surgeries, in outreach teams and specialist teams (e.g. drugs, alcohol and diabetes). There are teams on wards, outpatient departments, operating theatres, day surgeries – to name just a few. In the complex picture of the NHS, there are also teams within teams and individual members of staff may be members of many different teams, e.g. the consultant group, the operating team, the management team. Sometimes loyalties may be stretched or constrained so that the objectives of the different teams may pull the individual in different directions. The challenge of understanding these conflicts and their relation to patient outcomes and patient safety is considerable.

Despite the apparent importance of this field of study, there is relatively little hard evidence to date of the importance of teamworking and its indisputable impact on patient outcomes. In part, this is because the measurement of outcome is complex and many of those studies that have been conducted have used rather crude measures which have contributed to their lack of impact.

What is the evidence that team functioning affects patient safety?

There is a broad distinction to be made between patient outcomes and patient safety. There are numerous studies that have examined the impact of team functioning on general measures of patient outcome. There are fewer studies that look at the role of teams in the narrower concept of patient safety.

Some general benefits of teamworking have been demonstrated by Johnson and Johnson (1992). They conducted a meta-analysis of studies investigating the effects of team functioning versus individual performance and concluded that working in teams results in higher individual productivity on verbal, mathematical and procedural tasks. They also concluded that those working in teams show better self-esteem, psychological well-being and social support. If this pattern of effects derives from teamworking, it would be reasonable to conclude that high quality teamworking would lead to the kinds of changes which would improve patient outcomes and patient safety. Indeed, Shortell et al. (1994) found that intensive care units (ICUs) with team-orientated cultures, along with supportive nursing leadership, briefing, communication and collaborative approaches to problem solving, were significantly more efficient than other ICUs on measures of patient turnover. This study is particularly important since the size of the sample involved is very large. Data were collected on over a thousand patients from 42 ICUs. They measured the ICU performance via the risk adjusted mortality and length of stay measure (APACHE III), nurse turnover and technological facilities. They also collected 'climate' data from nurses, physicians, clerks and secretaries who completed the organizational inventory to assess communication patterns, problem solving and conflict management. Hence their conclusion that ICUs with a team-orientated culture and effective co-ordination are significantly more efficient and 'safe' in terms of moving patients into and out of the unit, is worth very careful consideration and worthy of evaluation in other settings.

A similar study that emphasizes the importance of interprofessional communication as a predictor of outcome/patient safety is that of Baggs et al. (1992). They hypothesized that patient risk as a consequence of transfer from ICU would be affected by the level of consultation between staff members and participating doctors and nurses about the decision to transfer. Fifty-six nurses and 31 doctors working on the unit were asked to rate the level of collaborative decision-making involved in the transfer of 286 patients. They found that the amount of interdisciplinary collaboration as reported by nurses was a significant predictor of successful transfer. Feiger and Schmitt (1979), working with an elderly population suffering from diabetes mellitus, found that the degree of participation of team members in team meetings, (which can be considered an indicator of team functioning), was related to positive outcomes for patients after a one-year period. These positive outcomes were expressed by assessing different functional abilities: social, physical, psychological and emotional. The team members consisted of nurses, nutritionists and physicians who devised individual care plans for each patient. Rubenstein et al. (1984) drew similar conclusions when they demonstrated that a team-based approach to the management of the elderly reduced morbidity and mortality.

Clearly we cannot conclude that the reduction in morbidity and mortality is necessarily because less 'errors' occurred but undoubtedly the overall safety of the patient has been influenced by the way the members of staff have interacted to deliver their care.

Effective teamworking has also been shown to influence outcomes for patients with mental health problems and substance abuse. We include consideration of this here since it raises the question as to what constitutes an 'error' in clinical areas where safe and effective 'treatment' or intervention is more psychosocially than physically based. In the mental health field the concept of an error is not as clear as it is in a surgical operating theatre. Yet decision-making errors or failure to perform at optimum levels can just as easily occur and affect patient outcomes and patient safety. If a patient's concerns are not adequately responded to by one or more members of a team, this may lead to non-compliance, or in extreme cases suicidal action. For example, Åberg-Wistedt et al. (1995) showed that schizophrenic patients randomly allocated to either team-based case management or standard psychiatric services required significantly fewer emergency visits and developed stronger social networks than those allocated to routine care.

Many studies which describe interventions aiming to improve patient safety, for example, evaluations of critical incident reporting procedures (e.g. Parke 2003) or evaluations of more efficient use of technology (e.g. Bumpus and al-Assaf 2003) conclude with a statement that continuing the improvement and maintaining changes will require improved teamwork and collaboration. So, implicit in many studies that do not directly address the 'teamwork' issue is the view that it will be an important component of a safer healthcare system.

All of these studies are in line with that of West et al. (2002) who report on a large-scale study of NHS organizations and concluded that there is a clear association between the percentage of staff who report working in teams and measures of patient mortality. If, as seems likely from this brief review, the quality of teamwork influences patient safety, the question then arises as to how best to teach teamworking skills and how to improve teamworking in clinical settings.

How can team functioning be improved?

There are some examples from the USA of studies that provide evidence that improvements in patient safety can be affected by interventions that improve team performance. One of the early American reports of the need to address multidisciplinary team communication if patient safety is to be improved is that of Connor et al. (2002) who describe the response taken by Boston's Cancer Institute to a medication error in 1995. They introduced a multidisciplinary team approach to identify and prevent errors and they included the patient and family members as an integral part of the team. This was seen as an important part of their error reduction strategy which also included a new chemotherapy order system, changing the culture from punitive to open discussion of errors and risks, as well as the introduction of a root cause analysis process for investigating near misses and errors.

Morey et al. (2002) report an evaluation of the 'Emergency Team Co-ordination Course' (ETCC), for clinical teams in Accident and Emergency departments (A&E). The ETCC was developed from looking at interventions developed in the aviation world where 'crew resource management' has become well established. They argued that hospital A&E departments share many of the same workplace characteristics of aviation crews: the stress, complex information, multiple players and high stake outcomes.

The basic principle that they adopted was that communication and co-ordination between staff members can be identified as discrete behaviours or events and that these can be taught where 'errors' in communication are observed. They developed an intervention, delivered by teams of instructors (one physician and one nurse) which was specially adapted for A&E situations.

This intervention included a number of physician–nurse pairs who acted as the instructors delivering a well-specified curriculum to mixed teams of emergency department staff (physicians, nurses and technicians). The curriculum involved a clear justification for looking at team functioning and an explanation of the difference between effective team functioning and more traditional 'work groups'. This intro-duction is followed by teaching modules which cover:

• team identification, leadership and conflict resolution;

• problem-solving strategies – how teams make decisions;

• communication and information exchange in teams;

• managing workload and performance management;

• improving team functioning by team performance reviews.

Morey et al. report a prospective multi-centre evaluation of this intervention using a quasi-experimental (untreated control group) design. The experimental group of 683 physicians, nurses and technicians shared significant improvement in quality of team behaviours, no change in subjective workload, but a reduction in clinical error rate. The experimental group also showed improved attitudes to teamwork and assessments of institutional support.

This is an important study since it describes an intervention and addresses the issues of cultural change that will be required for improvement to be maintained. Since it is a quasi-experimental study, it is not a definitive evaluation of the benefits of improving team functioning, and future evaluations will be needed to justify the significant resource that will be required to see such educational programmes adopted more widely. But it is a very important start and one that should be replicated in other clinical settings and other countries across the world.

In the UK, efforts are beginning to be made to develop similar programmes. A project at the Centre for Interprofessional Practice, University of East Anglia, involves developing and evaluating a team-based learning programme with certain similarities to that described by Morey et al. (2002). Specifically, it involves shared goal setting combined with conflict resolution and decision-making skills training. To date, 10 teams have undergone the programme, some are single site acute hospital teams, others are inter-agency teams concerned with child protection which span a number of agencies including health, social services, education and the police. The com-ponents of the team learning programme include: identification of goals for change, information sharing, conflict resolution and effective decision-making. These are all (apart from goal setting) similar to the USA ETCC programme.

Each team participates in five, two-hourly facilitated sessions. The intervention is being evaluated both quantitively and qualitatively. To date, significant improvements on all scales of the Anderson and West Team Climate Inventory (1994) are observed and some examples of changes in clinical practice that have a clear link to safety and risk reduction have been observed from the successful completion of the team identi-fied goals. Some of these are presented in Box 16.1.

Box 16.1 Successful changes to practice

- Introduction of a routine inhaler technique checking system for all patients on a respiratory medical ward.
- Improved patient education about stages of retinopathy and the importance of control of blood sugars.
- Improved junior doctors' completion of allergy information on drug charts through informal training by the ward pharmacist and senior doctor.
- Introduction of a risk analysis to determine order of priority for urgent cases awaiting angioplasty.
- Improved communication about patients' dietary needs, resulting in increased compliance with 'Nil by Mouth'.
- Minimized disruptions when doing drug rounds to improve efficiency and minimize risks of drug errors.
- Improved handover between the emergency assessment unit and the ward, leading to more accurate patient status information being transferred.
- Developing a process for reviewing critical incidents and near misses when protecting children in an acute trust hospital, and developing criteria for reporting incidents and a forum for presenting the information.

Future challenges

It is clear that the prevailing evidence to date suggests a link between team functioning and patient safety and suggests that interventions to improve team functioning may be effective in improving patient safety and reducing errors. However, we need considerably more evidence before we can be confident of this assertion and we should do all we can to encourage more research in this area.

Any evaluation or work in this area will need to take into account the fact that healthcare staff are often members of numerous teams and this multiple team membership may present conflict of loyalties which could make a committed contribution to a learning programme difficult. In addition, in the UK at present, a great deal of lip service is given to the notion of the multidisciplinary team but in many healthcare settings these so-called teams do not meet West's criteria for 'teams'. Many do not have clear leadership, membership or purpose. Hence before embarking on a team learning programme, being clear about the membership and the reality of their view of their 'teamliness' will be important.

In conclusion, it is important to recognize that patient safety is not just a consequence of individual action. All health professionals work in a complex environment in which the care of the patient is ultimately a consequence of the work and actions of a large number of different people. Patient safety may therefore be enhanced by improving a team's performance and not just an individual's performance. This chapter has considered specifically interprofessional team performance and has made some observations as to how to take this forward. Ultimately, the recognition of the importance of team functioning may lead to more sophisticated appraisal processes so that an individual's performance is appraised in the context of their team's performance. Examples of team appraisal can be found in other fields (US Office of Personnel Management 1998) and will be an important next step to consider as we attempt to consolidate improvements in team performance.

Box 16.2 Key points

- Patient care is delivered by groups of people, rarely by an individual alone.
- Patient outcomes are influenced by the quality of team functioning.
- The quality of teamworking in healthcare settings is not universally high.
- Evidence is growing that patient safety can be improved by interventions that teach teamworking skills to interprofessional groups.
- To maximize patient safety, effective teamworking will require cultural changes, including dissolution of 'old-fashioned demarcations' between healthcare professions as well as specific training in teamworking.

References

Åberg-Wistedt, A., Cresswell, T., Lidberg, Y., Liljenberg, B. and Osby, U. (1995) Two-year outcome of team-based intensive case management for patients with schizophrenia, *Psychiatric Services*, 46(12): 1263–6.

Anderson, N.R. and West, M.A. (1994) *The Team Climate Inventory: Manual and Users Guide*. Windsor: ASE Press.

Baggs, J.G., Ryan, S.A., Phelps, C.E., Richeson, J.F. and Johnson, J.E. (1992) The association between interdisciplinary collaboration and patient outcomes in a medical intensive care unit, *Journal of Acute and Critical Care*, 21(1): 18–24.

Baguley, P. (2002) *Teams and Team-Working*. London: Hodder and Stoughton.

Bumpus, L. and al-Assaf, A.F. (2003) Using performance improvement strategies to reduce and prevent medication errors, *Journal of Cardiovascular Management*, 14(6): 15–18.

Connor, M., Pont, P.R. and Conway, J. (2002) Multidisciplinary approaches to reducing error and risk in a patient care setting, *Crit Care Nurs Clin North Am.* 14(4): 359–67, viii.

Department of Health (2000a) *An Organization with a Memory*. London: The Stationery Office.

Department of Health (2000) *The NHS Plan*. London: The Stationery Office.

Feiger, S.M. and Schmitt, M.H. (1979) Collegiality in interdisciplinary health teams: its measurement and its effects, *Social Science and Medicine*, 13A: 217–29.

Johnson, D.W. and Johnson, R. (1992) *Positive Interdependence: The Heart of Cooperative Learning*. Edina, MN: Interaction Book Company.

Morey, J.C., Simon, R., Jay, G.D., Wears, R.L., Salisbury, M., Dukes, K.A. and Berns, S.D. (2002) Error reduction and performance improvement in the emergency department through formal teamwork training: evaluation results of the MedTeams Project, *Health Services Research*, 37(6): 1553–81.

Parke, T. (2003) Critical incident reporting in intensive care: experience in a District General Hospital, *Care of the Critically Ill*, 19(2): 42–4.

Rubenstein, L.Z., Josephson, K.R., Wieland, G.D., English, P.A., Sayre, M.S. and Kane, R.L. (1984) Effectiveness of a geriatric evaluation unit: a randomized clinical trial, *The New England Journal of Medicine*, 311(26): 1664–70.

Shortell, S.M., Zimmerman, J.E., Rousseau, D.M., Gillies, R.R., Wagner, D.P., Draper, E.A., Knaus, W.A. and Duffy, J. (1994) The performance of intensive care units: does good management make a difference? *Medical Care*, 32(5): 508–25.

Silén-Lipponen, M., Tossavainen, K., Turunen, H. and Smith, A. (2005) Potential errors and their prevention in operating room teamwork as experienced by Finnish, British and American nurses, *International Journal of Nursing Practice*, 11: 21–32.

United States Office of Personnel Management (1998) *Performance Appraisal for Teams: An Overview*. Washington, DC: Office of Personnel Management.

West, M.A., Borrill, C., Dawson, J., Scully, J., Carter, M., Anelay, S., Patterson, M. and Waring, J. (2002) The link between the management of employees and patient mortality in acute hospitals, *International Journal of Human Resource Management*, 13(8): 1299–310.

West, M.A. and Slater, J. (1996) *Teamworking in Primary Health Care: A Review of its Effectiveness*. London: Health Education Authority.

17
Conclusion – and the way forward
Ruth Boaden and Kieran Walshe

Each chapter in this book has made the case for the particular perspective it brings to patient safety to be a key part of research and development and has illustrated this with examples. Of itself, that is valuable in developing an evidence base for patient safety, but it is not enough – there are a number of other reasons why research into patient safety is important. The focus of the book has been on theory and research *into* practice – not just on theory, and each chapter has drawn on empirical studies in the area as well as highlighting areas for future work. Indeed, the third part of the book focussed on some case studies illustrating the process of putting theory into practice. This chapter brings together the themes of the book by discussing the context of patient safety and why it is important, the emerging research themes and the lessons learned to date from both research and practice.

The context: why patient safety research is important

Because it is about patients

Debates about the extent to which healthcare systems are really patient-centred have been raging for decades and will continue to do so. However, in the context of developing consumerism across the world, it is clear that the patient's role in healthcare provision is likely to continue to increase in importance. In the context of the NHS, which reflects wider international contexts in many ways, there is a clear policy aspiration for a 'patient-led NHS' (Department of Health 2005) with 'stronger standards and safeguards for patients' which contributes to the 'social imperative to make health care better and safer' (Stevens 2005). The introduction of patient choice in the UK, which has been a fundamental part of the system in the USA and other countries for many years, leads to an increased focus on safety as a key factor considered by patients when making a choice of healthcare provider.

However, although the study of safety should be patient-focussed, it is not a one-sided affair, applying only to those who provide health care. For many years those proposing frameworks for service quality have recognized that customer (patient) involvement in any service delivery process is a key determinant of overall quality and potential cause of variation in outcome (Desmet et al. 1998). The same can be said about patient safety – the best attempts of healthcare organizations to provide 'safe' services will be affected by the co-operation (or otherwise) of the patients themselves.

The data on the scale of harm caused by poor patient safety are described both in the introduction to this book and at various points throughout. Exposure to these mind-boggling statistics cannot fail to have an impact on anyone involved in health-care provision – and should prompt reflection on what could be done. The fact that all of us, and our families and friends, may also be patients at some point also provides an imperative for improving patient safety in our own spheres of influence. Patient safety is not only about patients – it is about us.

Because organizations are complex

The general complexity of healthcare provision means that 'simple improvement measures are seldom effective. The problems related to the improvement of patient care are large' (Grol et al. 2004: 3). They argue that any 'simple' approach to change management in the healthcare context is 'naïve and will fail' (2004: 3), a view supported by the patient safety literature (Lewis and Fletcher 2005). Any changes made to improve patient safety are within complex organizational contexts; this was brought out clearly in Chapter 2 by Liz West from the sociological perspective – who argued that organizational complexity makes healthcare vulnerable to breakdowns in communication – and in Chapter 13 by Sue Kirk and colleagues in their analysis of organizational culture. Several perspectives are explicit about errors being inevitable – in Chapter 1 Aneez Esmail argued that the practice of medicine is inherently unsafe and will always be so, and in Chapter 2 Liz West stated that the sociological perspec-tive regards errors as an inevitable, indeed normal, part of work. Although this perspective focuses on levels of analysis above the individual, others provided a com-plementary perspective on the role of the individual and the complexity that arises from their interaction within organizations; this was emphasized in Chapter 3 by Dianne Parker and Rebecca Lawton and in Chapter 16 by Shirley Pearce, Fiona Watts and colleagues. The balance between organizational and individual responsibil-ity for safety is one of the key themes of the book (see Introduction) and while there is a tension between these responsibilities, it is clear that both have a part to play in minimizing errors and the harm which may result from them, which is perhaps less inevitable.

Because safety and 'harm' are complex constructs

Research has an important role in identifying the nature, extent and context of 'harm' (Meyer and Eisenberg 2002), as well as uncovering the factors antecedent to injury, especially the underlying behavioural causes. Since understanding human thought and behaviour is the foundation of psychology, as described in Chapter 3 by Dianne Parker and Rebecca Lawton, there are useful contributions from this perspective to be made. The clinical perspective described in Chapter 1 by Aneez Esmail shows that there are a variety of patterns of thought and resultant behaviour which may depend on a wide range of factors, including professional training and background, and in

Chapter 14 Amanda Howe argued cogently that training can affect the way in which professionals behave in terms of safety. The assumption that safety will be enhanced because rules and guidelines are in place was explored in Chapter 15 by Tanya Claridge and colleagues and the systems and process perspective on safety was described as a development from quality management in Chapter 4 by Ruth Boaden, who pointed out the minimal impact of many quality improvement approaches because they were too focussed on systems rather than individuals and the interaction between them.

Because safety interventions are complex

Developing and understanding interventions designed to reduce error are a key role for research (Meyer and Eisenberg 2002) and when technology is a part of this, as described in Chapter 5 by Paul Beatty, such interventions may be even more complex despite their laudable aims. This also complicates the research and evaluation processes required to generate evidence about the efficacy of such interventions.

Issues concerning the extent of transferability of safety frameworks and interventions are another key theme of this book (see Introduction) and one which requires a deeper understanding of the complexity of the interventions. Just because a particular approach appears to have improved safety in e.g. the airline industry, to what extent should we assume that it will also 'work' in health care? This theme is touched on by many chapters in this book:

- In Chapter 1 Aneez Esmail was clear that research from other areas has not made its way far enough into the practice of medicine.

- In Chapter 3 Dianne Parker and Rebecca Lawton described how psychology has contributed to improving safety in a variety of industries, and how health care could learn from this.

- In Chapter 4 Ruth Boaden described lessons learned from the implementation of quality management and their implications for patient safety.

- In Chapter 8 Sally Giles, Maureen Baker and colleagues highlighted the lessons that can be learned about effective incident reporting systems from other high risk industries.

- In Chapter 13 Sue Kirk and colleagues discussed the variability of culture assessment tools in terms of their transferability to healthcare settings.

- In Chapter 15 Tanya Claridge, Dianne Parker and colleagues described how other industries have lessons to teach health care about how to develop and implement rules to maximize compliance.

- In Chapter 9 Tony Avery and colleagues also highlighted that there is learning to be had from other countries and healthcare settings when the use of large databases and chart review is being considered.

Emerging research themes

The scope of topics and approaches covered in this book means that a huge variety of themes have been identified as requiring further research. The scale of research into patient safety is growing rapidly (Thomson and Carthey 2004) with the Agency for Healthcare Research and Quality (AHRQ) in the USA receiving $50 million for research in patient safety in 2001/2. The World Health Organization (WHO) launched its World Alliance for Patient Safety (WAPS), in October 2004, to advance the patient safety goal 'First do no harm' and cut the number of illness, injuries and death suffered by patients. Research in the UK is being promoted by the NHS National Patient Safety Agency (NPSA) and specifically through its Patient Safety Research Programme (PSRP), currently with an annual budget of £1.5 million. The NPSA Research Strategy (Thomson and Carthey 2004) shows that their objectives are to work with others to build world-wide capacity in patient safety research, identifying and filling gaps in knowledge, and avoiding duplication of effort, although they have yet to identify specific areas of work.

Themes for research are clearer if located within an overall framework which takes into account the development of patient safety as a field, something echoed in the details of the WHO WAPS by the identification of a number of stages of development:

1. *Developing a recognition of safety:* 'some level of sensitization to the harm that can occur within health care systems'.[1] While it could be argued that this has already been achieved in most Western countries, this is not the case in many others.

2. *Understanding when adverse events occur:* 'assess the nature and incidence of adverse outcomes'. There is clearly more research to be done in this area, but on its own this does nothing to actually improve patient safety. This area was also identified as important in the UK (Department of Health 2000) and described there as 'establishing the size and nature of the problem'.

3. *Understanding what causes adverse events:* 'it is also essential to understand the causes of adverse outcomes, which may vary according to country, health care system and treatment or procedure'. It is this stage which has occupied the resources of many researchers to date, as shown in Part 2 of this book. This step is one where the contributions of a variety of disciplines, especially those not traditionally within the boundaries of medicine, are valuable, as this book shows. It is also the stage at which the complexities of human behaviour, not only on an individual basis but in terms of their interaction within organizations, become a key focus of research activity.

4. *Developing methods of preventing adverse events:* which may involve piloting before widespread implementation. This will also involve evaluation and assessment of the effects of the interventions, which will be complex due to the complexity of both safety and safety interventions. The issues of prevention may also be addressed by systems design; poor system design can of itself be a cause of error 'every system is perfectly designed to achieved the results it achieves' (Berwick 1996).

5. *Ensuring that change is sustained in both individuals and organizations*: although this was not explicitly described by the WHO, this factor was identified by Department of Health (2000) and is not unique to patient safety, applying instead to all areas of organizational change (Burnes 2004).

There have been a few studies of existing patient safety research, which also highlight areas for future study, with the most comprehensive being Cooper et al. (2001) for the US National Patient Safety Foundation and Westwood et al. (2005) for the NPSA, and the study from a user perspective undertaken by Meyer and Eisenberg (2002). The major themes that emerge from these studies and the research reported in this book are discussed now. At the end of each topic, the key areas emerging as having future research potential are summarized.

Understanding when adverse events occur

This was a key theme of a number of chapters in this book:

- In Chapter 7 Sue Dovey, John Hickner and colleagues provided a clear review of the ways in which adverse events can be categorized and emphasize that such frameworks are able to enhance understanding, rather than simply classifying data. As such frameworks develop, and a small number of widely accepted ones emerge, data will become more comparable and lessons will be more transferable.

- In Chapter 8, Sally Giles, Maureen Baker and colleagues showed how incident reporting has the potential to promote learning and improve safety.

- Another perspective on considering the occurrence of adverse events was provided in Chapter 9 by Tony Avery and colleagues in describing how large databases and chart review are used to study medical error, although they acknowledge that, on their own, such studies do not provide sufficient clinical information to judge the presence of error.

The theme of one perspective being helpful but not sufficient was also covered in the two chapters that focus on legal aspects of patient safety, and one which was identified as important by Cooper et al. (2001). In Chapter 6 Michael Jones clearly described what the legal perspective can contribute – a forensic investigation into what went wrong and allocating responsibility for that – although it is not good at identifying organizational issues that hamper patient safety. Claims review was described in Chapter 11 by Charles Vincent and colleagues, who highlighted the biases and limitations of this method, but also the contribution that it can make when combined with other methods. It is clear that this area of study has not yet been exhausted, and the potential cost implications of litigation will undoubtedly mean that it remains an important area for future study.

This area was described by Meyer and Eisenberg (2002) as the 'epidemiology of errors' from the user perspective and is an area where there is still much to be done. The use of tools from other areas (as described in Chapter 4 by Ruth Boaden) can be helpful in analysing this, although their use alone does not constitute improvement in patient safety. In particular, just as there is a continuing requirement to measure quality of care, so there is also a need to identify what the key indicators of safety are, and this is an area still to be developed. The recent adoption by the NHS of a new performance framework (Department of Health 2004) which has as one of its key domains 'patient safety' is likely to accelerate the importance of this area, at least in the UK, but there is scope for more research here. This area is also linked to the increasing requirement for public disclosure of safety information (Cooper et al. 2001), something which can draw on the lessons from the use of taxonomies of errors, as described in Chapter 7 by Sue Dovey, John Hickner and colleagues.

Economics is linked to both the occurrence of adverse events, and their consequences. To date, this has not been a major focus of patient safety research and the frameworks developed in quality management around the cost of quality, and the cost of prevention are not currently well developed in the patient safety field. A recent paper for the UK NPSA (Gray 2005) has reviewed existing studies in this area, and it is expected that this will generate new research. To date, there appears to be little research showing that patient safety interventions reduce costs; in Chapter 6 Michael Jones cited the lack of empirical evidence to support the intuitive assumption that improved patient safety will reduce the cost of litigation. This suggests that the causal link between safety and outcomes may be much more complex than this, a conclusion supported by the sociological perspective described in Chapter 2 by Liz West.

Areas for future research

- the legal aspects of patient safety;
- the development of common taxonomies of error;
- indicators of patient safety;
- public disclosure of safety data;
- the economics of safety.

Understanding what causes adverse events

Much of the research reported in this book focusses on this step and, it is hoped, makes a valuable contribution to the development of this understanding. For example, in Chapter 10 Steve Rogers and colleagues covered the issues concerned with the analysis of critical incidents, which is one way to develop this understanding. This area (i.e. 'basic understanding about the causes of error and systems failure') has been reported as being under-represented by Cooper et al. (2001).

One aspect of this is communication and information-sharing, especially between organizations (Cooper et al. 2001), something which it is hoped will be enabled by national organizations like the NPSA. Communication between individuals is also a feature highlighted by perspectives in this book; in Chapter 2 Liz West described the impact of individuals communicating primarily with those like themselves, which creates barriers between groups hampering the development of patient safety.

Another aspect concerns the technical issues around automation, medical devices and other physical issues (Cooper et al. 2001), something which was covered here in

Chapter 5 by Paul Beatty. The area of health informatics is a vast area for development, in the NHS through Connecting for Health[2] and in other countries through similar systems. The lack of a national health infrastructure in the USA means that this area is not as well developed on a national scale, however. The role of technology in general, in both causing and helping to address adverse events, is a key theme for future research. In Chapter 5 Paul Beatty was clear that on its own, a technological approach will never provide a total 'solution' to patient safety issues and he suggests that there is enormous potential when it is combined with the human factors approach.

'Human factors' were covered by a number of chapters in this book:

- In Chapter 16, Shirley Pearce, Fiona Watts and colleagues showed that there is evidence that effective team working does make a difference to patient safety.
- In Chapter 12, Rachel Finn and Justin Waring demonstrated that the ethnographic approach can show how teamwork practices emerge from the multi-professional cultures within healthcare.
- The psychological perspective described in Chapter 3 by Dianne Parker and Rebecca Lawton showed that the most useful taxonomies of error are those based on human error theory.
- In Chapter 4 Ruth Boaden showed that the failure of quality management initiatives was often attributed to lack of attention to the 'people factors'.

The concept of culture as the shared beliefs, norms and values of the individuals within an organization, as described in Chapter 13 by Sue Kirk and colleagues in terms of patient safety, and in Chapter 12 by Rachel Finn and Justin Waring in terms of the potential contribution of the ethnographic approach, is increasingly cited as important in improving patient safety. This draws on perspectives relating to individuals, and has been relatively under-represented in earlier research (Cooper et al. 2001; Meyer and Eisenberg 2002). Calls for changes in environment and culture are numerous (Lewis and Fletcher 2005) as claims are made that developing an effective safety culture is important to make lasting changes to patient safety (see Chapter 13). These two chapters were both clear that their approaches do not provide total solutions, but are best used along with other tools and measures, because of the nebulous and multidimensional nature of safety culture.

Areas for future research

- analysing incidents after the event for causal factors;
- communication and information-sharing;
- the impact of health informatics on patient safety;
- the 'human dimensions' at the individual and organizational (cultural) level.

Developing methods of preventing adverse events

Involving patients themselves in improving safety was a key factor identified in the study by Cooper et al. (2001) and the rationale for this is described in the first section of this chapter. There appears to be little, if any, research already completed in this area (Westwood et al. 2005) and this is the reason why this has not been a major feature of this book although in Chapter 9 Tony Avery and colleagues described how interviews with patients may enhance the method of chart review and in Chapter 14 Amanda Howe concluded that culture change could be achieved by shifting the balance of power to patients. This is the area with perhaps the most potential for future development. One of the future challenges of this aspect is the ethics of research in general, which has not been given significant consideration in patient safety research to date.

One area of importance in the prevention of adverse events may be that of education and training, raised from the user perspective in Meyer and Eisenberg (2002) and covered in Chapter 14 by Amanda Howe – where it was argued that safety has to be part of both the formal training process and the safety culture of the training organization. Apart from learning through formal programmes, there are, however, many other areas where learning can occur in order to progress patient safety; in Chapter 3 Dianne Parker and Rebecca Lawton claimed that utilizing the psychological approach to patient safety facilitates organizational learning, as did Sally Giles, Maureen Baker and colleagues when discussing incident reporting in Chapter 8, where they made it clear that continuous learning, analysis and action are needed to lead to safer care.

In Chapter 5 Paul Beatty described the limitations of 'engineering out' human error through the use of technology, i.e. attempting to solve error before it happens but this is problematic, not only in engineering terms but also from the human perspective. He proposes that the use of persuasive technologies in future may enable behaviour change. In order to prevent adverse events occurring, we need, however, to ensure that research is carried out both during and after the 'event': much research in patient safety to date has been 'after the event' and focussed on understanding when adverse events have occurred (in the past). However, to understand more fully the organizational and behavioural factors which impact patient safety, it is necessary to carry out more prospective and concurrent research, a point argued in Chapter 12 by Rachel Finn and Justin Waring. The use of chart review, as described in Chapter 9 by Tony Avery and colleagues, could benefit from prospective studies and the use of claims analysis as described in Chapter 11 by Charles Vincent and colleagues could also be enhanced by more standardized data collection methods and formats designed in advance.

Another aspect of the development of preventative methods is the need to provide evidence for interventions, rather than simply a hunch that they may work. This links not only to views on appropriate research methodologies for the development of such evidence, but also to the transferability of interventions from other sectors, something which has been a key theme of this book, and lacking in earlier research reviews (Cooper et al. 2001). There are a few studies in this area, reviewed by Westwood et al. (2005), with the main types of studies including automation in medication dispensing (referred to by Paul Beatty in Chapter 5), evaluation of training programmes (referred to in Chapter 14 by Amanda Howe), studies of attitude towards error and its reporting (as described in Chapter 3 by Dianne Parker and Rebecca Lawton) and the effectiveness of adverse event reporting systems (covered in Chapter 8 by Sally Giles and colleagues). However, this list is hardly comprehensive in its coverage of the areas of potential improvement in patient safety and illustrates the areas still to be researched effectively.

The need for 'evidence' is often most clearly articulated by clinical professionals – who tend to be uncertain of the status of rules they are required to follow (as described in Chapter 15 by Tanya Claridge and colleagues) and are not comfortable with providing care according to rules. Their adherence to rules, or otherwise, is also put under scrutiny when litigation is undertaken, as described by Michael Jones in Chapter 6. This professional perspective was also articulated by Aneez Esmail in Chapter 1, who stated that the depth of uncertainty in the practice of medicine – sometimes presenting itself as a need for 'more' or 'better' evidence – is not easily understood by those outside the profession. Steve Rogers claimed, in Chapter 10, that training is needed for professionals in incident investigation if it is to be effective. Clearly the role of professionals, and their behaviour, are key areas for future research.

The role of financial incentives in improving patient safety is discussed by Lewis and Fletcher (2005) within the context of overall health policy and it is argued that the 'business case' for patient safety will become more prominent in the UK as it moves to a more pluralistic provider system, as well as mobilizing commitment from healthcare organizations. However, using incentives is not straightforward, especially if they are not carefully aligned with 'negative' incentives, and it can be difficult to predict what the impact of incentives will be on the whole system. There may be a need for financial incentives at the level of the 'health community' as well as the individual healthcare provider institutions if gains are to be realized. Policy dynamics, especially those concerned with financial incentives, are key drivers of organization behaviour in every area, including patient safety, even where individuals within the organization would be happy to agree that 'safer = better'.

Areas for future research

- patient involvement in improving safety;
- education and training of healthcare provider staff;
- the development of a coherent evidence base for interventions;
- the role and contribution of professionals in improving patient safety;
- the role of financial incentives in improving patient safety.

Ensuring that change is sustained in both individuals and organizations

Sustaining change is often described as making something 'mainstream' and it can be argued that patient safety will only be effectively improved when it is mainstreamed into all areas of healthcare activity. This applies to research – where safety, like economics, should be a part of any research application and project – but in Chapter 14 Amanda Howe made the same argument for safety being a part of every training programme, rather than a bolt-on extra, and being a part of the organizational culture. Consideration of the context of the organization will also be an influencing factor on patient safety – as described by Liz West in Chapter 2 and Rachel Finn and Justin Waring in Chapter 12. The key role of organizational (and safety) culture was described:

- in Chapter 13 by Sue Kirk and colleagues as contributing to making lasting improvements in patient safety;
- in Chapter 8 by Sally Giles and colleagues as important in incident reporting systems being effective;
- in Chapter 4 by Ruth Boaden, when describing studies in the field of quality management;
- in Chapter 14 by Amanda Howe who summarized the position as follows: 'patient safety is a topic for a new kind of learning – one that puts the patient first, the learner second, our failures in the open, and our humility to the test – a true "learning culture" '.

However, this can lead to a tension between those keen to promote patient safety as a 'new' field of study – something separate although linked to other more established fields – and those who wish it to be mainstreamed and totally integrated. This tension is evident in some of the literature about patient safety, as it was in the field of quality management. However, Lewis and Fletcher (2005) are clear that the integration of patient safety 'into the routine measurement, monitoring, review and improvement of everyday healthcare practice' is an 'over-riding goal' of UK patient safety strategy and they justify this because they believe it is the only way to achieve large-scale change. Linking patient safety to the routine of healthcare provision may be enhanced by more research into the use of routine data for patient safety improvement – rather than requiring new data sources and methods of data collections. However, as discussed in the following section, this can only be done with a clear understanding of the policy context and the levers for change that follow from the health policy adopted.

Areas for future research

- the mechanisms of mainstreaming patient safety;
- how an effective culture for safety can be developed;
- the role of the policy context in sustaining change.

What has been learned

The multidisciplinary theme of this book has shown that there are a number of lessons to be learned, all of which have future implications. While some are more applicable to healthcare practitioners and others to those carrying out research from the academic domain, these lessons need to be understood by all those involved in patient safety if improvements are to be made.

This is only the beginning

It is rare that any field of study will claim to have 'enough' evidence, but the scope of patient safety means that there are still many areas where there is little research of any substance. This is clear by the research activities of the national organizations promoting patient safety, which are well established in the USA, Australia and the UK, and each has a research programme, as well as the information given throughout this book. This is good news for those whose 'business' is carrying out such research and should also lead to good news for patients themselves in terms of safer health care if the research fulfils its aims, although as Liz West pointed out in Chapter 2, there is little evidence at present to link social organization and adverse events, so such an outcome is not automatic.

However, even where research does exist, it is not always 'good' research – not only in terms of patient safety research but also in terms of quality improvement and change in general. A useful summary of 'the relatively few well-conducted empirical studies' of change management within the NHS (Iles and Sutherland 2001) cites a few evaluation studies on TQM and BPR (Joss and Kogan 1995; Packwood et al. 1998; McNulty and Ferlie 2002) but reiterates the lack of research that considers the factors that shape organizational change in the NHS. Variations in study design in safety research – often poorly described – with the field dominated by observational and survey studies was noted by Westwood et al. (2005) in their review focussed entirely on original research studies. They concluded that the studies lacked focus, with most being small-scale – single hospital or groups of units – which leads to difficulties in generalizing the results. There is, however, a recognition that the prevalence of case reports and before-and-after papers may be able to disseminate results more quickly than research using other methods which takes longer to conduct, and the same can be argued for patient safety. Concerns about the quality of evidence – particularly from clinical professionals – may be well founded and need to be addressed if research is to have credibility and applicability.

There is no coherent field of study in patient safety as yet, and although it may be that some believe that safety should be mainstreamed as soon as possible without the need for separation, this is not a universal view. The academic field of quality and safety is developing more quickly than some other fields traditionally have done (Stevens 2005) because of its social imperative although its development may also be hampered by the research designs used: 'weak designs . . . do not allow internally valid conclusions and the consequence is that the science of quality improvement will proceed ineffectively in healthcare' (Speroff and O'Connor 2004). Research in the area of quality improvement is often criticized for being anecdotal rather than systematic and independently evaluated: 'measures and programmes to change practice are more often implemented on the basis of firm beliefs' (Grol et al. 2004) and this will in turn affect the development of the field of study: 'A science is only as good as its research methods' (Grol et al. 2004: 129). It is not currently clear whether those involved should be pursuing the establishment of a patient safety field of study or discipline, or whether their over-riding concern should be to simply get the results of their endeavours applied in practice.

The context is important

An important outcome from the increased involvement of a wider range of disciplines in patient safety research has been the emphasis on organizations and their context. The Introduction to this book made the case for further consideration of the organizational dimensions of patient safety, as have a number of authors of chapters in this book. This is not to downplay the contribution of those who study issues at an individual level, but this is not going to be sufficient to develop a fuller understanding of the complex issue of patient safety and the ways in which it can be improved; the sociological perspective described in Chapter 2 by Liz West provides evidence that environmental pressures can deflect organizations from their main goals. Even at the level of individual approaches to patient safety, such as the use of quality improvement techniques as described by Ruth Boaden in Chapter 4, taxonomies of error as described in Chapter 7 by Sue Dovey and colleagues, and incident reporting as described in Chapter 8 by Sally Giles and colleagues, the circumstances in which they are used will determine their effectiveness. While some claim that this issue is now widely accepted as important – 'poor quality and unsafe care, we have come to understand, are caused by faulty systems and not by faulty individuals and no single group is to blame' (Moss 2003) – this acceptance is not always translated into the research that is carried out, or the implications that follow from it. The challenge to researchers and practitioners is to consider the wider issues in any research they carry out, or any results that are implemented to improve patient safety.

However, there is also the wider national and international context which will impact on the study and practice of patient safety. A recent account of the development of a national patient safety strategy (Lewis and Fletcher 2005) stresses the importance of understanding the policy context, since this 'creates the conditions that facilitate or hinder the achievement of policy objectives'. In the USA it is clear that professionalism (as described by Aneez Esmail in Chapter 1), regulation (including the use of rules, as described by Tanya Claridge, Dianne Parker and colleagues in Chapter 15) and markets can all be used to prompt safer actions by hospitals (Devers et al. 2004), and the main influencing factors on progress (Wachter 2004) are described as regulation, error reporting systems, information technology, the US malpractice system and workforce and training issues. However, it is argued (Lewis and Fletcher 2005) that in a less pluralistic system such as the UK, there are additional factors including measurement and system-wide learning, purchasing and design, organizational governance and development, the NHS infrastructure and public and patient involvement, all of which are likely to have more impact in a 'national' health system like that of the UK. Current strategy in the UK involves system-wide learning, the use of purchasing strategies to maximize the use of safer healthcare products, incorporating safety into facility design and work with patients to increase their influence over safety through national involvement mechanisms.

Even identifying these 'levers' for change is not sufficient on its own – it is the interaction between them that requires further investigation, especially where there are apparent contradictions. For example, what is the appropriate balance between external incentives such as regulation and internal factors like the strengthening of the professional ethos of clinicians to increase the motivation to improve (Lewis and Fletcher 2005)? There is an emerging evidence base (some of which was described in Chapter 15 by Tanya Claridge and colleagues) about this which has a lot to contribute to the overall study of patient safety, and which is likely to be the topic of much future health policy research.

Multidisciplinary research has methodological challenges

What constitutes good research is an eternal matter of debate, it is widely acknowledged, and is a tenet of this book, that patient safety requires a multidisciplinary approach to research and therefore a variety of methods will be needed – the qualitative vs quantitative debate is not one to be had here and whether there ever can, or should be, an 'optimal methodology' (Grol et al. 2004) is not considered here. This book shows that no one perspective or set of tools is sufficient – and this has been acknowledged both implicitly and explicitly by the authors of most of the chapters in this book.

Analysis of research designs suitable for use in healthcare quality improvement makes the point that 'quality improvement is typically conducted in settings where random allocation to groups is not possible for ethical reasons or where the environmental condition prevents experimenter manipulation' (Speroff and O'Connor 2004) although this statement is true for many other types of management-led initiatives too (Lilford et al. 2003). The assumption that experimental design is the most appropriate for this type of study is also challenged by many, especially those from a social science perspective and can be linked to the debate on evidence-based management (Walshe and Rundall 2001; Hewison 2004), contrasting with the evidence-based medicine view (Sackett et al. 1996). The range of methods that might be used is vast and some of the ones not explicitly covered in this book include experimental design, action research, systematic reviews and evaluation research *per se*.

This book has shown that multidisciplinary research is not only desirable but necessary in order to provide the richness of information needed to develop understanding of why things go wrong and how this may be improved. If multidisciplinary research means that 'people bring separate theories, skills, data, and ideas to bear on a common problem' (Golde and Gallagher 1999), in practice, this is likely to mean studies with multiple method designs, where researchers actively communicate and share ideas and approaches as well as data throughout the research process (rather than simply reporting results from different methods in different sections of a final report) as well as making coherent and consistent efforts to triangulate results from various methods and provide a rich picture of the outcomes. This is not a call for interdisciplinary research ('bringing together people and ideas from different disciplines to jointly frame a problem, agree on a methodological approach, and analyse the data') (Golde et al. 1999) because the challenges of the process might outweigh the rewards and there are pragmatic reasons for getting on with patient safety research in order to lead to improvements in practice as soon as possible.

This is a challenge to those working in academic systems where reward appears to be given in disciplinary silos rather than for multidisciplinary work, something already noted in reviews of patient safety research: 'The literature is still scattered and diverse, partly because of its inherent multidisciplinary nature' (Thomson and Carthey 2004).

Research needs to make a difference

This is a theme throughout the book – research needs to make a difference for patients – and it may be that it is best placed to do this by the integration of patient safety as a consideration as part of the fabric of healthcare provision. More research on the stages of 'understanding what causes adverse events' and 'developing interventions to improve patient safety' is clearly needed and that knowledge then needs to be utilized.

The Introduction to this book raised the question of how far healthcare organizations might have to go to even compare in terms of safety with other industries. The evidence in this book has shown that there are methods and approaches available to support this progress, and that catching up with others is probably not the ultimate aim. The key focus of healthcare provision has to be about patients: it will be down to those providing health care to utilize this evidence and these approaches to make a practical difference for patients, showing that 'knowledge about "what to do" has at last been translated into significant actions that truly make a difference for patients' (Moss 2004).

Notes

1 http://www.who.int/patientsafety/research/en/
2 Known before 1 April 2005 as the NHS National Programme for IT (www.npfit.nhs.uk).

References

Berwick, D. M. (1996) A primer on leading the improvement of systems, *British Medical Journal*, 312(7031): 619–22.

Burnes, B. (2004) *Managing Change*. Harlow: Pearson Education.

Cooper, J.B., Sorensen, A.V., Anderson, S.M., Zipperer, L.A., Blum, L.N. and Blim, J.F. (2001) *Current Research on Patient Safety in the United States*. Chicago: National Patient Safety Foundation.

Department of Health (2000) *Building a Safer NHS for Patients: Implementing An Organization with a Memory*. London: The Stationery Office.

Department of Health (2004) *Standards for Better Health: Health Care Standards for Services under the NHS*. London: The Stationery Office.

Department of Health (2005) *Creating a Patient-led NHS: Delivering the NHS Improvement Plan*. London: The Stationery Office.

Desmet, S., Looy, B.V. and Dierdonck, R.V. (1998) The nature of services, in B.V. Looy, R.V. Dierdonck and P. Gemmel (eds) *Services Management: An Integrated Approach*. London: Financial Times/Prentice Hall.

Devers, K.J., Hoangmai, H.P. and Gigi, L. (2004) What is driving hospitals' patient safety efforts? *Health Affairs*, 23(2): 103–16.

Golde, C.M. and Gallagher, H.A. (1999) The challenges of conducting interdisciplinary research in traditional doctoral programmes, *Ecosystems*, 2(4): 281–5.

Gray, A. (2005) *Adverse Events and the National Health Service: An Economic Perspective.* London: National Patient Safety Agency.

Grol, R., Baker, R. and Moss, F. (eds) (2004) *Quality Improvement Research: Understanding the Science of Change in Health Care.* London: BMJ Books.

Hewison, A. (2004) Evidence-based management in the NHS: is it possible? *Journal of Health Organization and Management*, 18(4/5): 336–48.

Iles, V. and Sutherland, K. (2001) *Organizational Change: A Review for Health Care Managers, Professionals and Researchers.* London: NHS Co-ordinating Centre for NHS Service Delivery and Organisation R&D.

Joss, R. and Kogan, M. (1995) *Advancing Quality: Total Quality Management in the NHS.* Buckingham: Open University Press.

Lewis, R.Q. and Fletcher, M. (2005) Implementing a national strategy for patient safety: lessons from the National Health Service in England, *Quality and Safety in Health Care*, 14(2): 135–9.

Lilford, R., Dobbie, F., Warren, R., Braunholtz, D. and Boaden, R. (2003) Top rate business research: has the emperor got any clothes? *Health Services Management Research*, 16(3): 147–54.

McNulty, T. and Ferlie, E. (2002) *Reengineering Health Care: The Complexities of Organizational Transformation.* Oxford: Oxford University Press.

Meyer, G.S. and Eisenberg, J.M. (2002) The end of the beginning: the strategic approach to patient safety research, *Quality and Safety in Health Care*, 11: 3–4.

Moss, F. (2003) Working differently for better, safer care, *Quality and Safety in Health Care*, 12:90001 1i–.

Moss, F. (2004) The clinician, the patient and the organization: a crucial three-sided relationship, *Quality and Safety in Health Care*, 13(6): 406–7.

Packwood, T., Pollitt, C. and Roberts, S. (1998) Good medicine? A case study of business process re-engineering in a hospital, *Policy and Politics*, 26(4): 401–15.

Sackett, D.L., Rosenberg, W.M.C., Gray, J.A.M., Haynes, R.B. and Richardson, W.S. (1996) Evidence based medicine: what it is and what it isn't, *British Medical Journal*, 312(7023): 71–2.

Speroff, T. and O'Connor, G.T. (2004) Study designs for PDSA quality improvement research, *Quality Management in Health Care*, 13(1): 17–32.

Stevens, D.P. (2005) Three questions for QSHC, *Quality and Safety in Health Care*, 14(1): 2–3.

Thomson, R. and Carthey, J. (2004) *Research and Development Strategy.* London: National Patient Safety Agency.

Wachter, R.M. (2004) The end of the beginning: patient safety five years after *To Err Is Human, Health Affairs – Web Exclusive*, W4-534–W4-545.

Walshe, K. and Rundall, T.G. (2001) Evidence-based mnagement: from theory to practice in health care, *The Milbank Quarterly*, 79(3): 429–57.

Westwood, M., Rodgers, M. and Snowden, A. (2005) *Patient Safety: A Mapping of the Research Literature, Draft Report.* London: National Patient Safety Agency.

Index